PREVENTING ALCOHOL ABUSE

PREVENTING ALCOHOL ABUSE

Alcohol, Culture, and Control

David J. Hanson

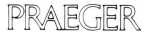

Westport, Connecticut
London

Library of Congress Cataloging-in-Publication Data

Hanson, David J.
  Preventing alcohol abuse : alcohol, culture, and control / David
J. Hanson.
    p.   cm.
  Includes bibliographical references and index.
  ISBN 0–275–94926–5 (alk. paper)
  1. Alcoholism. 2. Alcoholism—Prevention. 3. Drinking of
alcoholic beverages. I. Title.
  HV5035.H25   1995
  362.29′27—dc20   94–37889

British Library Cataloguing in Publication Data is available.

Library of Congress Catalog Card Number: 94–37889
ISBN: 0–275–94926–5

First published in 1995

Praeger Publishers, 88 Post Road West, Westport, CT 06881
An imprint of Greenwood Publishing Group, Inc.

Printed in the United States of America

The paper used in this book complies with the
Permanent Paper Standard issued by the National
Information Standards Organization (Z39.48–1984).

10 9 8 7 6 5 4 3

Copyright Acknowledgments

The author and the publisher gratefully acknowledge permission to use the following:

Excerpts from "An Assessment of the Effects of Alcohol Ordinances on Selected Behaviors and Conditions," by R. Thomas Dull and David J. Giacopassi in *Journal of Drug Issues*. Copyright 1986. Used with the permission of *Journal of Drug Issues*.

Excerpts from "Formal and Informal Social Control over Drinking," by Ira H. Cisin in John A. Ewing and Beatrice A. Rouse. (eds.) *Drinking: Alcohol in American Society—Issues and Current Research*. Copyright 1978, Nelson-Hall, Chicago, IL. Used with the permission of Nelson-Hall Publishers.

Excerpts from *Primitive Drinking: A Study of the Uses and Functions of Alcohol in Preliterate Societies* by Chandler Washburne. College and University Press, New York. Copyright 1961. Used with the permission of the author.

Excerpts from *Primary Prevention of Alcohol Abuse and Alcoholism: An Evaluation of the Control of Consumption Policy* by David J. Pittman. Social Science Institute, Washington University, St. Louis, MO. Copyright 1980. Used with the permission of the author.

Table 3.1 reprinted from J.F. Lotterhos, E.D. Glover, D. Holbert, and R.C. Barnes, "Intentionality of College Students Regarding North Carolina's 21-year Drinking Age Law," in *International Journal of the Addictions* 23, Marcel Dekker Inc., NY, 1988. Used with the permission of Marcel Dekker Inc.

To

Carol and Cynthia

Contents

Illustrations

Preface

This book reflects the influence of my mentor, Dr. Ephraim H. Mizruchi of Syracuse University, who has had a major impact on my intellectual development. Also more important than she probably realizes has been the long and very fruitful alcohol research collaboration that Dr. Ruth C. Engs of Indiana University and I share.

The data retrieval skills of Holly Chambers and the interlibrary loan services of Kathy LaClair, both of Potsdam College's Crumb Library, greatly facilitated this research and are much appreciated.

Pivotal to the entire writing effort was Jackie Rush, whose consistent patience, attention to detail, sound judgment and good humor were invaluable.

Introduction

Alcoholic beverages play important roles in enhancing life among peoples around the world and have done so throughout history. Most societies use alcohol with few problems, although in some the consequences of drinking are viewed as a cause of public concern. The cross-cultural evidence indicates that drinking abuse will be low in any group in which drinking customs, values and sanctions are clear, agreed upon by all, consistent with other customs of the group and characterized by prescriptions for moderate drinking and proscriptions against immoderate drinking (Blacker, 1966, p. 68). While prohibition in the United States and elsewhere has proven to be a failure, the simplistic prohibitionist impulse is found today in the controversial control-of-consumption approach, which seeks to increase abstinence and to reduce the average per capita consumption of alcohol. This is in spite of extensive evidence that the moderate consumption of alcohol is associated with the lower incidence of heart and other disease and with greater longevity. There is little evidence that control-of-consumption policies are effective in reducing heavy consumption or the problems associated with it. If these policies should prove to be effective in reducing consumption among moderate and light drinkers, this very success may have negative consequences for the vast majority of drinkers without any offsetting positive effect among the minority of drinkers who consume heavily. Such a trade-off is unacceptable. Therefore, understandings based on the cross-cultural and scientific evidence yield recommendations that the current control-of-consumption attack upon alcohol should be ended; that all attempts to stigmatize alcohol as a "dirty drug," as a poison, as inherently harmful, or as a substance to be abhorred and shunned should be ended; that governmental agencies formulate and implement policies that incorporate the concept of moderate or responsible drinking along with the choice of abstinence; that systematic efforts be made to clarify and emphasize the distinctions between acceptable and unacceptable drinking; that unacceptable drinking behaviors be strongly sanctioned, both legally and socially; that parents be permitted to serve alcohol to their offspring of any age, not only at home, but in restaurants, parks, and other locations under their direct control and supervision; and that educational efforts encourage moderate use of alcohol among those who choose to drink.

The desire to manipulate and control the behavior of others seems endemic to humans. "Regardless of how often it fails or leads us in destructive directions, the search for simple solutions to complex problems seems endlessly appealing" (Lazar and Ford, 1977, p. 29). Nowhere is this more apparent than in the control-of-consumption program of questionable legislation to restrict the consumption of alcohol. Like the prohibitionists earlier in the century, whom they so closely resemble, the neo-drys of today are convinced that they have found the solution to reducing alcohol problems. Unfortunately, their simplistic approach is not only of questionable value but is potentially dangerous to the health and longevity of the typical drinker.

REFERENCES

Blacker, Edward. Sociocultural factors in alcoholism. *International Psychiatry Clinics*, 1966, *3*, pp. 51-80.

Lazar, Irving, Ford, John. Untitled reaction of review panel. In: Lauderdale, Michael L. An Analysis of the Control Theory of Alcoholism. Denver, CO: Education Commission of the States, 1977, pp. 29-34.

1

A Look Back

Alcohol is a valued product which has provided important functions for people throughout all history. From the earliest times to the present, alcohol has played an important role in religion and worship. Historically, alcoholic beverages have served as sources of needed nutrients and have been widely used for their medicinal, antiseptic, and analgesic properties. The role of such beverages as pleasing thirst quenchers is obvious and they play an important role in enhancing the enjoyment and quality of life. They can be a social lubricant, can facilitate relaxation, can provide pharmacological pleasure, and can increase the pleasure of eating. Thus, while alcohol has always been misused by a minority of drinkers, it has clearly proved to be beneficial to most.

ANCIENT PERIOD

While no one knows when beverage alcohol was first used, it was presumably the result of a fortuitous accident that occurred at least tens of thousands of years ago. However, the discovery of late Stone Age beer jugs has established the fact that intentionally fermented beverages existed at least as early as the Neolithic period (cir. 10,000 B.C.) (Patrick, 1952, pp. 12-13), and it has been suggested that beer may have preceded bread as a staple (Braidwood et al., 1953; Katz and Voigt, 1987); wine clearly appeared as a finished product in Egyptian pictographs around 4,000 B.C. (Lucia, 1963a, p. 216). The earliest alcoholic beverages may have been made from berries or honey (Blum et al., 1969, p. 25; Roueché, 1960, p. 8; French, 1890, p. 3) and wine making may have originated in the wild grape regions of the Middle East. Oral tradition recorded in the Old Testament (Genesis 9:20) asserts that Noah planted a vineyard on Mt. Ararat in what is now Turkey. In Sumeria, beer and wine were used for medicinal purposes as early as 2,000 B.C. (Babor, 1986, p. 1).

Brewing dates from the beginning of civilization in ancient Egypt (Cherrington, 1925, v. 1, p. 404) and alcoholic beverages were very important in that country. Symbolic of this is the fact that while many gods were local or familial, Osiris, the god of wine, was worshiped throughout the entire country (Lucia, 1963b, p. 152). The Egyptians believed that this important god also invented beer (King, 1947, p. 11), a beverage that was considered a necessity of life; it was brewed in the home "on an everyday basis" (Marciniak, 1992, p. 2). Both beer and wine were deified and offered to gods. Cellars and wine presses even had a god whose hieroglyph was a wine press (Ghaliounqui, 1979, p. 5). The ancient Egyptians made at least seventeen varieties of beer and at least 24 varieties of wine (Ghaliounqui, 1979, pp. 8 and 11). Alcoholic beverages were used for pleasure, nutrition, medicine, ritual, remuneration (Cherrington, 1925, v. 1, p. 405) and funerary purposes. The latter involved storing the beverages in tombs of the deceased for their use in the after-life (King, 1947, p. 11; Darby, 1977, p. 576).

Numerous accounts of the period stressed the importance of moderation, and these norms were both secular and religious (Darby, 1977, p. 58). While Egyptians did not generally appear to define inebriety as a problem, they warned against taverns (which were often houses of prostitution) and excessive drinking (Lutz, 1922, pp. 97, 105-108). After reviewing extensive evidence regarding the widespread but generally moderate use of alcoholic beverage, the historian Darby makes a most important observation: all these accounts are warped by the fact that moderate users "were overshadowed by their more boisterous counterparts who added 'color' to history" (Darby, 1977, p. 590). Thus, the intemperate use of alcohol throughout history receives a disproportionate amount of attention. Those who abuse alcohol cause problems, draw attention to themselves, are highly visible and cause legislation to be enacted. The vast majority of drinkers, who neither experience nor cause difficulties, are not noteworthy. Consequently, moderation is largely ignored by observers and writers.

Beer was the major beverage among the Babylonians, and as early as 2,700 B.C. they worshiped a wine goddess and other wine deities (Hyams, 1965, pp. 38-39). Babylonians regularly used both beer and wine as offerings to their gods (Lutz, 1922, pp. 125-126). Around 1,750 B.C., the famous Code of Hammurabi devoted attention to alcohol. However, there were no penalties for drunkenness; in fact, it was not even mentioned. The concern was fair commerce in alcohol (Popham, 1978, pp. 232-233). Nevertheless, although it was not a crime, it would appear that the Babylonians were critical of drunkenness (Lutz, 1922, pp. 115-116).[1]

A variety of alcoholic beverages have been used in China since prehistoric times (Granet, 1957, p. 144). Alcohol was considered a spiritual (mental) food rather than a material (physical) food, and extensive documentary evidence attests to the important role it played in the religious life (Hucker, 1975, p. 28; Fei-Peng, 1982, p. 13). "In ancient times people always drank when holding a memorial ceremony, offering sacrifices to gods or their ancestors, pledging resolution before going into battle, celebrating victory, before feuding and official executions, for taking an oath of allegiance, while attending the ceremonies of birth, marriage, reunions, departures, death, and festival banquets" (Fei-Peng, 1982, p. 13).

A Chinese imperial edict of about 1,116 B.C. makes it clear that the use of alcohol in moderation was believed to be prescribed by heaven. Whether or not it was prescribed by heaven, it was clearly beneficial to the treasury. At the time of Marco Polo (1254?-1324?) it was drunk daily (Gernet, 1962, p. 139) and was one of the treasury's biggest sources of income (Balazs, 1964, p. 97).

Alcoholic beverages were widely used in all segments of Chinese society, were used as a source of inspiration, were important for hospitality, were an antidote for fatigue, and were sometimes misused (Samuelson, 1878, pp. 19-20, 22, 26-27; Fei-Peng, 1982, p. 137; Simoons, 1991, pp. 448-459). Laws against making wine were enacted and repealed forty-one times between 1,100 B.C. and A.D. 1,400. (Alcoholism and Drug Addiction Research Foundation of Ontario, 1961, p. 5). However, a commentator writing around 650 B.C. asserted that people "will not do without beer. To prohibit it and secure total abstinence from it is beyond the power even of sages. Hence, therefore, we have warnings on the abuse of it" (quoted in Roueché, 1963, p. 179; similar translation quoted in Samuelson, 1878, p. 20).

While the art of wine making reached the Hellenic peninsula by about 2,000 B.C. (Younger, 1966, p. 79), the first alcoholic beverage to obtain widespread popularity in what is now Greece was mead, a fermented beverage made from honey and water. However, by 1,700 B.C., wine making was commonplace, and during the next thousand years wine drinking assumed the same function so commonly found around the world: It was incorporated into religious rituals, it became important in hospitality, it was used for medicinal purposes and it became an integral part of daily meals (Babor, 1986, pp. 2-3). As a beverage, it was drunk in many ways: warm and chilled, pure and mixed with water, plain and spiced (Raymond, 1927, p. 53).

Contemporary writers observed that the Greeks were among the most temperate of ancient peoples. This appears to result from their rules stressing moderate drinking, their praise of temperance, their practice of diluting wine with water, and their avoidance of excess in general (Austin, 1985, p. 11). An exception to this ideal of moderation was the cult of Dionysus, in which intoxication was believed to bring people closer to their deity (Sournia, 1990, pp. 5-6; Raymond, 1927, p. 55).

While habitual drunkenness was rare, intoxication at banquets and festivals was not unusual (Austin, 1985, p. 11). In fact, the symposium, a gathering of men for an evening of conversation, entertainment and drinking typically ended in intoxication (Babor, 1986, p. 4). However, while there are no references in ancient Greek literature to mass drunkenness among the Greeks, there are references to it among foreign peoples (Patrick, 1952, p. 18). By 425 B.C., warnings against intemperance, especially at symposia, appear to become more frequent (Austin, 1985, pp. 21-22).

Xenophon (431-351 B.C.) and Plato (429-347 B.C.) both praised the moderate use of wine as beneficial to health and happiness, but both were critical of drunkenness, which appears to have become a problem. Hippocrates (cir. 460-370 B.C.) identified numerous medicinal properties of wine, which had long been used for its therapeutic value (Lucia, 1963a, pp. 36-40). Later, both Aristotle (384-322 B.C.) and Zeno (cir. 336-264 B.C.) were very critical of drunkenness (Austin, 1985, pp. 23, 25, and 27).

Among Greeks, the Macedonians viewed intemperance as a sign of masculinity and were well-known for their drunkenness. Their king, Alexander the Great (336-323 B.C.), whose mother adhered to the Dionysian cult, developed a reputation for inebriety (Sournia, 1990, pp. 8-9; Babor, 1986, p. 5).

The Hebrews were reportedly introduced to wine during their captivity in Egypt. When Moses led them to Canaan (Palestine) around 1,200 B.C., they are reported to have regretted leaving behind the wines of Egypt (Numbers 20:5); however, they found vineyards to be plentiful in their new land (Lutz, 1922, p. 25). Around 850 B.C., the use of wine was criticized by the Rechabites and Nazarites,[2] two conservative nomadic groups who practiced abstinence from alcohol (Lutz, 1922, p. 133; Samuelson, 1878, pp. 62-63).

In 586 B.C., the Hebrews were conquered by the Babylonians and deported to Babylon. However, in 539 B.C., the Persians captured the city and released the Hebrews from their Exile (Daniel 5: 1-4). Following the Exile, the Hebrews developed Judaism as it is now known, and they can be said to have become Jews. During the next 200 years, sobriety increased and pockets of antagonism to wine disappeared. It became a common beverage for all classes and ages, including the very young; an important source of nourishment; a prominent part in the festivities of the people; a widely appreciated medicine; an essential provision for any fortress; and an important commodity. In short, it came to be seen as a necessary element in the life of the Hebrews (Raymond, 1927, p. 23). While there was still opposition to excessive drinking, it was no longer assumed that drinking inevitably led to drunkenness. Wine came to be seen as a blessing from God and a symbol of joy (Psalms 104; Zachariah 10:7). These changes in beliefs and behaviors appear to be related to a rejection of belief in pagan gods, a new emphasis on individual morality, and the integration of secular drinking behaviors into religious ceremonies and their subsequent modification (Austin, 1985, pp. 18-19; Patai, 1980, pp. 61-73; Keller, 1970, pp. 290-294). Around 525 B.C., it was ruled that the *kiddush* (pronouncement of the Sabbath) should be recited over a blessed cup of wine. This established the regular drinking of wine in Jewish ceremonies outside the Temple (Austin, 1985, p. 19).

King Cyrus of Persia frequently praised to his people the virtue of the moderate consumption of alcohol (cir. 525 B.C.). However, ritual intoxication appears to have been used as an adjunct to decision making and, at least after his death, drunkenness was not uncommon (Austin, 1985, p. 19).

Between the founding of Rome in 753 B.C. until the third century B.C., there is consensus among historians that the Romans practiced great moderation in drinking (Austin, 1985, p. 17). After the Roman conquest of the Italian peninsula and the rest of the Mediterranean basin (509 to 133 B.C.), the traditional Roman values of temperance, frugality and simplicity were gradually replaced by heavy drinking, ambition, degeneracy and corruption (Babor, 1986, p. 7; Wallbank & Taylor, 1954, p. 163). The Dionysian rites (*Bacchanalia*, in Latin) spread to Italy during this period and were subsequently outlawed by the Senate (Lausanne, 1969, p. 4; Cherrington, 1925, v. 1, pp. 251-252).

Practices that encouraged excessive drinking included drinking before meals on an empty stomach, inducing vomiting to permit the consumption of more food and wine, and drinking games. The latter included, for example, rapidly consuming as many cups as indicated by a throw of the dice (Babor, 1986, p. 10).

By the second and first centuries B.C., intoxication was no longer a rarity, and most prominent men of affairs (for example, Cato the Elder and Julius Caesar) were praised for their moderation in drinking. This would appear to be in response to growing misuse of alcohol in society, because before that time temperance was not singled out for praise as exemplary behavior. As the republic continued to decay, excessive drinking spread and some, such as Marc Antony (d. 30 B.C.), even took pride in their destructive drinking behavior (Austin, 1985, pp. 28 and 32-33).

EARLY CHRISTIAN PERIOD

With the dawn of Christianity and its gradual displacement of the previously dominant religions, the drinking attitudes and behaviors of Europe began to be influenced by the New Testament (Babor, 1986, p. 11). The earliest biblical writings after the death of Jesus (cir. A.D. 30) contain few references to alcohol. This may have reflected the fact that drunkenness was largely an upper-status vice with which Jesus had little contact (Raymond, 1927, pp. 81-82). Austin (1985, p. 35) has pointed out that Jesus used wine (Matthew 15:11; Luke 7:33-35) and approved of its moderate consumption (Matthew 15:11). On the other hand, he severely attacked drunkenness (Luke 21:34, 12:42; Matthew 24:45-51). The later writings of St. Paul (d. 64?) deal with alcohol in detail and are important to Christian doctrine on the subject. He considered wine to be a creation of God and therefore inherently good (1 Timothy 4:4), recommended its use for medicinal purposes (1 Timothy 5:23), but consistently condemned drunkenness (1 Corinthians 3:16-17, 5:11, 6:10; Galatians 5:19-21; Romans 13:3) and recommended abstinence for those who could not control their drinking.[3]

However, late in the second century, several heretical sects rejected alcohol and called for abstinence. By the late fourth and early fifth centuries, the Church responded by asserting that wine was an inherently good gift of God to be used and enjoyed. While individuals may choose not to drink, to despise wine was heresy. The Church advocated its moderate use but rejected excessive or abusive use as a sin. Those individuals who could not drink in moderation were urged to abstain (Austin, 1985, pp. 44 and 47-48).

It is clear that both the Old and New Testaments are clear and consistent in their condemnation of drunkenness. However, some Christians today argue that whenever "wine" was used by Jesus or praised as a gift of God, it was really grape juice; only when it caused drunkenness was it wine. Thus, they interpret the Bible as asserting that grape juice is good and that drinking it is acceptable to God but that wine is bad and that drinking it is unacceptable. This reasoning appears to be incorrect for at least two reasons. First, neither the Hebrew nor Biblical Greek word for wine can be translated or interpreted as referring to grape juice. Secondly, grape juice would quickly ferment into wine in the warm climate of the Mediterranean region without refrigeration or modern methods of preservation (Royce, 1986, pp. 55-56; Raymond, 1927, pp. 18-22; Hewitt, 1980, pp. 11-12).

The spread of Christianity and of viticulture in Western Europe occurred simultaneously (Lausanne, 1969, p. 367; Sournia, 1990, p. 12). Interestingly, St. Martin of Tours (316-397) was actively engaged in both spreading the Gospel and planting vineyards (Patrick, 1952, pp. 26-27).

In an effort to maintain traditional Jewish culture against the rise of Christianity, which was converting numerous Jews (Wallbank & Taylor, 1954, p. 227), detailed rules concerning the use of wine were incorporated into the Talmud. Importantly, wine was integrated into many religious ceremonies in limited quantity (Spiegel, 1979, pp. 20 -29; Raymond, 1927, 45-47). In the social and political upheavals that rose as the fall of Rome approached in the fifth century, concern grew among rabbis that Judaism and its culture were in increasing danger.[4] Consequently, more Talmudic rules were laid down concerning the use of wine. These included the amount of wine that could be drunk on the Sabbath, the way in which wine was to be drunk, the legal status of wine in any way connected with idolatry, and the extent of personal responsibility for behavior while intoxicated (Austin, 1985, pp. 36 and 50).

Roman abuse of alcohol appears to have peaked around mid-first century (Jellinek, 1976, pp. 1,736-1,739). Wine had become the most popular beverage, and as Rome attracted a large influx of displaced persons, it was distributed free or at cost (Babor, 1986, pp. 7-8). This led to occasional excesses at festivals, victory triumphs and other celebrations, as described by contemporaries. The four emperors who ruled from A.D. 37 to A.D. 69 were all known for their abusive drinking. However, the emperors who followed were known for their temperance, and literary sources suggest that problem drinking decreased substantially in the Empire. Although there continued to be some criticisms of abusive drinking over the next several hundred years, most evidence indicates a decline of such behavior (Austin, 1985 pp. 37-44, p. 46, pp. 48-50). The fall of Rome and the western Roman Empire occurred in 476 (Wallbank and Taylor, 1954, pp. 220-221).

Around A.D. 230, the Greek scholar Athenaeus wrote extensively on drinking and advocated moderation. The extensive attention to drinking, famous drinks, and drinking cups (of which he described 100) reflected the importance of wine to the Greeks (Austin, 1985, pp. 45-46).

THE MIDDLE AGES

The Middle Ages, that period of approximately one thousand years between the fall of Rome and the beginning of the High Renaissance (cir. 1500), saw numerous developments in life in general and in drinking in particular. In the early Middle Ages, mead, rustic beers, and wild fruit wines became increasingly popular, especially among Celts, Anglo-Saxons, Germans, and Scandinavians. However, wines remained the beverage of preference in the Romance countries (what is now Italy, Spain and France) (Babor, 1986, p. 11).

With the collapse of the Roman Empire and decline of urban life, religious institutions, particularly monasteries, became the repositories of the brewing and winemaking techniques that had been earlier developed (Babor, 1986, p. 11). While rustic beers continued to be produced in homes, the art of brewing essentially became the province of monks, who carefully guarded their knowledge (Cherrington, 1925, v. 1, p. 405). Virtually all beer of good quality was brewed by monks until the twelfth century. Around the thirteenth century, hops (which both flavors and preserves) became a common ingredient in some beers, especially in northern Europe (Wilson, 1991, p. 375).[5] Ale, often a thick and nutritious soupy beverage, soured quickly and was made for local consumption (Austin, 1985, p. 54, pp. 87-88).

Not surprisingly, the monasteries also maintained viticulture. Importantly, they had the resources, security, and stability in that often turbulent time to improve the quality of their vines slowly over time (Seward, 1979, pp. 15 and 25-35). The monks also had the education and time necessary to enhance their viticultural skills (Lichine, 1974, p. 3). Throughout the Middle Ages, the best vineyards were owned and tended by the monasteries, and *vinum theologium* was considered superior to others (Patrick, 1952, p. 27). In addition to making wine necessary to celebrate the mass, the monasteries also produced large quantities to support the maintenance and expansion of the monastic movement (Babor, 1986, p. 11). While most wine was made and consumed locally, some wine trade did continue in spite of the deteriorating roads (Hyams, 1965, p. 151; Wilson, 1991, p. 371).

By the millennium, the most popular form of festivities in England were known as "ales," and both ale and beer were at the top of lists of products to be given to lords for rent. As towns were established in twelfth-century Germany, they were granted the privilege of brewing and selling beer in their immediate localities. A flourishing artisan brewing industry developed in many towns, about which there was strong civic pride (Cherrington, 1925, v. 1, p. 405; Austin

1985, pp. 68, 74, 82-83).

The most important development regarding alcohol throughout the Middle Ages was probably that of distillation. Interestingly, considerable disagreement exists concerning who discovered distillation and when the discovery was made.[6] However, it was Albertus Magnus (1193-1280) who first clearly described the process which made possible the manufacture of distilled liquors (Patrick, 1952, p. 29). Knowledge of the process began to spread slowly among monks, physicians and alchemists, who were interested in distilled alcohol as a cure for ailments. At that time it was called *aqua vitae*, "water of life,"[7] but was later known as brandy. The latter term was derived from the Dutch *brandewijn*, meaning burnt (or distilled) wine (Seward, 1979, p. 151; Roueché, 1963, pp. 172-173).

The Black Death and subsequent plagues, which began in the mid-fourteenth century, dramatically changed people's perception of their lives and place in the cosmos. With no understanding or control of the plagues that reduced the population by as much as 82% in some villages, "processions of flagellants mobbed city and village streets, hoping, by the pains they inflicted on themselves and each other, to take the edge off the plagues they attributed to God's wrath over human folly" (Slavin, 1973, pp. 12-16). Some dramatically increased their consumption of alcohol in the belief that this might protect them from the mysterious disease, while others thought that through moderation in all things, including alcohol, they could be saved. It would appear that, on balance, consumption of alcohol was high. For example, in Bavaria, beer consumption was probably about 300 liters per capita a year (compared to 150 liters today) and in Florence wine consumption was about ten barrels per capita a year. Understandably, the consumption of distilled spirits, which was exclusively for medicinal purposes, increased in popularity (Austin, 1985, pp. 104-105, 107-108).

As the end of the Middle Ages approached, the popularity of beer spread to England, France and Scotland (Austin, pp. 118-119). Beer brewers were recognized officially as a guild in England (Monckton, 1966, pp. 69-70), and the adulteration of beer or wine became punishable by death in Scotland (Cherrington, 1929, vol. 5, p. 2,383). Importantly, the consumption of spirits as a beverage began to occur (Braudel, 1974, p. 171).

EARLY MODERN PERIOD

The early modern period was generally characterized by increasing prosperity and wealth. Towns and cities grew in size and number, foreign lands were discovered and colonized, and trade expanded. Perhaps more importantly, there developed a new view of the world. The medieval emphasis on other-worldliness--the belief that life in this world is only a preparation for heaven--slowly gave way, especially among the wealthy and well educated, to an interest in life in the here and now (Wallbank & Taylor, 1954, p. 513).

The Protestant Reformation and rise of aggressive national states destroyed the ideal of a universal Church overseeing a Holy Roman Empire. Rationality, individualism, and science heavily impacted the prevalent emotional idealism, communalism, and traditional religion (Wallbank & Taylor, 1954, pp. 513-518; Slavin, 1973, ch. 5-7).

However, the Protestant leaders such as Luther, Calvin, the leaders of the Anglican Church and even the Puritans did not differ substantially from the teachings of the Catholic Church: alcohol was a gift of God and created to be used in moderation for pleasure, enjoyment and health; drunkenness was viewed as a sin (Austin, 1985, p. 194).

From this period through at least the beginning of the eighteenth century, attitudes toward drinking were characterized by a continued recognition of the positive nature of moderate consumption and an increased concern over the negative effects of drunkenness. The latter, which was generally viewed as arising out of the increased self-indulgence of the time, was seen as a threat to spiritual salvation and societal well-being. Intoxication was also inconsistent with the emerging emphasis on rational mastery of self and world and on work and efficiency (Austin, 1985, pp. 129-130).

However, consumption of alcohol was often high. In the sixteenth century, alcohol beverage consumption reached 100 liters per person per year in Valladolid, Spain, and Polish peasants consumed up to three liters of beer per day (Braudel, 1974, pp. 236-238). In Coventry, the average amount of beer and ale consumed was about 17 pints per person per week, compared to about three pints today (Monckton, 1966, p. 95); nationwide, consumption was about one pint per day per capita. Swedish beer consumption may have been 40 times higher than in modern Sweden. English sailors received a ration of a gallon of beer per day, while soldiers received two-thirds of a gallon. In Denmark, the usual consumption of beer appears to have been a gallon per day for adult laborers and sailors (Austin, 1985, pp. 170, 186, 192).

However, the production and distribution of spirits spread slowly. Spirit drinking was still largely for medicinal purposes throughout most of the sixteenth century. It has been said of distilled alcohol that "the sixteenth century created it; the seventeenth century consolidated it; the eighteenth popularized it" (Braudel, 1967, p. 170).

A beverage that clearly made its debut during the seventeenth century was sparkling champagne. The credit for that development goes primarily to Dom Pérignon, the wine-master in a French abbey. Around 1668, he used strong bottles, invented a more efficient cork (and one which could contain the effervescence in those strong bottles), and began developing the technique of blending the contents. However, another century would pass before problems, especially bursting bottles, would be solved and sparkling champagne would become popular (Younger, 1966, pp. 345-346; Doxat, 1971, p. 54; Seward, 1979, pp. 139-143).

The original grain spirit, whiskey, appears to have first been distilled in

Ireland. While its specific origins are unknown (Magee, 1980, p. 7; Wilson, 1973, p. 7) there is evidence that by the sixteenth century it was widely consumed in some parts of Scotland (Roueché, 1963, pp. 175-176). It was also during the seventeenth century that Franciscus Sylvius (or Franz de la Boë), a professor of medicine at the University of Leyden, distilled spirits from grain. To mask the raw spirit taste, then considered objectionable, it was generally flavored with juniper berries. The resulting beverage was known as *junever*, the Dutch word for "juniper." The French changed the name to *geniévre*, which the English changed to "geneva" and then modified to "gin"[8] (Roueché, 1963, pp. 173-174). Originally used for medicinal purposes, the use of gin as a social drink did not grow rapidly at first (Doxat, 1972, p. 98; Watney, 1976, p. 10). However, in 1690, England passed "An Act for the Encouraging of the Distillation of Brandy and Spirits from Corn" and within four years the annual production of distilled spirits, most of which was gin, reached nearly one million gallons (Roueché, 1963, p. 174).

The seventeenth century also saw the Virginia colonists continue the traditional belief that alcoholic beverages are a natural food and are good when used in moderation. In fact, beer arrived with the first colonists, who considered it essential to their well-being (Baron, 1962, pp. 3-8). The Puritan minister Increase Mather preached in favor of alcohol but against its abuse: "Drink is in itself a good creature of God, and to be received with thankfulness, but the abuse of drink is from Satan; the wine is from God, but the Drunkard is from the Devil" (quoted in Rorabaugh, 1979, p. 30). During that century the first distillery was established in the colonies on what is now Staten Island (Roueché, 1963, p. 178), cultivation of hops began in Massachusetts, and both brewing and distilling were legislatively encouraged in Maryland (Austin, 1985, pp. 230 and 249).

Rum is produced by distilling fermented molasses, which is the residue left after sugar has been made from sugar cane. Although it was introduced to the world, and presumably invented, by the first European settlers in the West Indies, no one knows when it was first produced or by what individual. But by 1657, a rum distillery was operating in Boston. It was highly successful and within a generation the manufacture of rum would become colonial New England's largest and most prosperous industry (Roueché, 1963, p. 178).

The dawn of the eighteenth century saw Parliament pass legislation designed to encourage the use of grain for distilling spirits. In 1685, consumption of gin had been slightly over one-half million gallons (Sournia, 1990, p. 20). By 1714, gin production stood at two million gallons (Roueché, 1963, p. 174). In 1727, official (declared and taxed) production reached five million gallons; six years later the London area alone produced eleven million gallons of gin (French, 1890, p. 271; Samuelson, 1878, pp. 160-161; Watney, 1976, p. 16). The English government actively promoted gin production to utilize surplus grain and to raise revenue. Encouraged by public policy, very cheap spirits flooded the market at a time when there was little stigma attached to drunkenness and when the growing urban poor in London sought relief from the new-found insecurities and harsh realities of urban life (Watney, 1976, p. 17; Austin, 1985, pp. xxi-xxii). Thus developed the so-called Gin Epidemic. While the negative effects of that phenomenon may have been exaggerated[9] (Sournia, 1990, p. 21; Mathias, 1959, p. xxv), Parliament passed legislation in 1736 to discourage consumption by prohibiting the sale of gin in quantities of less than two gallons and raising the tax on it dramatically.[10] However, the peak in consumption was reached seven years later, when the nation of six and one-half million people drank over 18 million gallons of gin. And most was consumed by the small minority of the population then living in London and other cities; people in the countryside largely remained loyal to beer, ale and cider (Doxat, 1972, pp. 98-100; Watney, 1976, p. 17).

After its dramatic peak, gin consumption rapidly declined. From 18 million gallons in 1743, it dropped to just over seven million gallons in 1751 and to less than two million by 1758, and generally declined to the end of the century (Ashton, 1955, p. 243). A number of factors appear to have converged to discourage consumption of gin. These include the production of higher quality beer of lower price, rising corn prices and taxes which eroded the price advantage of gin, a temporary ban on distilling, a stigmatization of drinking gin, an increasing criticism of drunkenness, a newer standard of behavior that criticized coarseness and excess, increased tea and coffee consumption, an increase in piety and increasing industrialization with a consequent emphasis on sobriety and labor efficiency (Sournia, 1990, p. 22; King, 1947, p. 117; Austin, 1985, pp. xxiii-xxiv, 324-325, 351; Younger, 1966, p. 341).

While drunkenness was still an accepted part of life in the eighteenth century (Austin, 1985, p. xxv), the nineteenth century would bring a change in attitudes as a result of increasing industrialization and the need for a reliable and punctual work force (Porter, 1990, p. xii). Self-discipline was needed in place of self-expression, and task orientation had to replace relaxed conviviality. Drunkenness would come to be defined as a threat to industrial efficiency and growth.

Problems commonly associated with industrialization and rapid urbanization were also attributed to alcohol. Thus, problems such as urban crime, poverty and high infant mortality rates were blamed on alcohol, although "it is likely that gross overcrowding and unemployment had much to do with these problems" (Sournia, 1990, p. 21). Over time, more and more personal, social and religious/moral problems would be blamed on alcohol. And not only would it be enough to prevent drunkenness; any consumption of alcohol would come to be seen as unacceptable. Groups that began by promoting temperance--the moderate use of alcohol--would ultimately become abolitionist and press for the complete and total prohibition of the production and distribution of beverage alcohol. Unfortunately, this would not eliminate social problems but would compound the situation by creating additional problems. But more about that later.

SUMMARY AND CONCLUSION

It is clear that alcohol has been highly valued and in continuous use by peoples throughout history. Reflecting its vital role, consumption of alcohol in moderation has rarely been questioned throughout most of recorded time. To the contrary, "Fermented dietary beverage, and especially wine, was so common an element in the various cultures that it was taken for granted as one of the basic elements of survival and self-preservation" (Lucia, 1963b, p. 165). Indicative of its value is the fact that it has frequently been acceptable as a medium of exchange. For example, in Medieval England, ale was often used to pay toll, rent or debts (Watney, 1974, p. 16).

From the earliest times alcohol has played an important role in religion,[11] typically seen as a gift of deities and closely associated with their worship. Religious rejection of alcohol appears to be a rare phenomenon. When it does occur, such rejection may be unrelated to alcohol per se, but reflect other considerations. For example, the nomadic Rechabites rejected wine because they associated it with an unacceptable agricultural life style. Nazarites abstained only during the period of their probation, after which they returned to drinking (Sournia, 1990, p.5; Samuelson, 1878, pp. 62-63). Among other reasons, Mohammed may have forbidden alcohol in order further to distinguish his followers from those of other religions (Royce, 1986, p. 57).

Alcoholic beverages have also been an important source of nutrients and calories (Braudel, 1974, p. 175). In ancient Egypt, the phrase "bread and beer" stood for all food and was also a common greeting. Many alcoholic beverages, such as Egyptian *bouza* and Sudanese *merissa*, contain high levels of protein, fat and carbohydrates, a fact which helps explain the frequent lack of nutritional deficiencies in some populations whose diets are generally poor. Importantly, the levels of amino acids and vitamins increase during fermentation (Ghaliounqui, 1979, pp. 8-9). While modern food technology uses enrichment or fortification to improve the nutrition of foods, it is possible to achieve nutritional enrichment naturally through fermentation (Steinkraus, 1979, p. 36).

Alcoholic beverages have long served as thirst quenchers. Water pollution is far from new; to the contrary, supplies have generally been either unhealthful or questionable at best. Ancient writers rarely wrote about water, except as a warning (Ghaliounqui, 1979, p. 3). Travelers crossing what is now Zaire in 1648 reported having to drink water which resembled horse's urine. In the late eighteenth century most Parisians drank water from a very muddy and often chemically polluted Seine (Braudel, 1967, pp. 159-161). Coffee and tea were not introduced into Europe until the mid-seventeenth century, and it was another hundred or more years before they were commonly consumed on a daily basis (Austin, 1985, pp. 251, 254, 351, 359, 366).

Another important function of alcohol has been therapeutic or medicinal. Current research suggests that the moderate consumption of alcohol is preferable to abstinence. It appears to reduce the incidence of coronary heart disease (e.g.,

Razay, 1992; Jackson et al., 1991; Klatsky et al., 1990, p. 745; Rimm et al., 1991; Miller et al., 1990), cancer (e.g., Bofetta and Garfinkel, 1990) and osteoporosis (e.g., Gavaler and Van Thiel, 1992), among many other diseases and conditions, and to increase longevity (e.g., DeLabry et al., 1992). It has clearly been a major analgesic, and one widely available to people in pain. Relatedly, it has provided relief from the fatigue of hard labor.

Not to be underestimated is the important role alcohol has served in enhancing the enjoyment and quality of life. It can serve as a social lubricant, can provide entertainment, can facilitate relaxation, can provide pharmacological pleasure and can facilitate gustatory satisfaction. With regard to the last point, it should be noted, "The enjoyment of a good meal can be greatly enhanced by beer or wine. The taste of foods may be perceived with greater enjoyment when wine or beer accompanies a meal, perhaps from a solvent action which prevents persistent contact of the food with the taste organs, or perhaps only from the contrasting taste of the beer or wine and the food" (Gastineau et al., 1979, p. xx).

While alcohol has always been misused by a minority of drinkers, it has clearly proved to be beneficial to most. In the words of a former Director of the National Institute on Alcohol Abuse and Alcoholism, ". . . alcohol has existed longer than all human memory. It has outlived generations, nations, epochs and ages. It is a part of us, and that is fortunate indeed. For although alcohol will always be the master of some, for most of us it will continue to be the servant of man" (Chafetz, 1965, p. 223).

NOTES

1. For additional information on alcohol among the Babylonians, see Lutz (1922, pp. 115-133).

2. Individuals could choose to consecrate themselves to God for a period of time and become Nazarites, after which time they could again drink wine (Numbers 6:1-4; Numbers 6:13-20; Speigel, 1979, pp. 12-13).

3. For additional documentation on the views of Jesus and the early church see Hewitt (1980, pp. 14-19) and Raymond (1927, pp. 27-91). For references to alcohol in the Old Testament categorized into positive and negative and into realms (physical, psychological, social, religious or economic), see O'Brien and Seller (1982).

4. Christianity became the sole and official religion of the Roman Empire in 395 A.D. (Wallbank and Taylor, 1954, p. 230).

5. While hops may have been used in Bavaria as early as around the mid-eighth century, exactly when and where brewing with hops began is unclear (Mathias, 1959, p. 4; Cherrington, 1925, v.1, p. 405). However, hopped beer was actually "a new drink altogether, a product of the technique of precise fermentation using only barley, and in which addition of hops ensured an agreeable taste and the possibility of better conservation" (Claudian, 1970, p. 10; Austin, 1985, p. 87). It might be noted that old recipes added such ingredients as "poppy seeds, mushrooms, aromatics, honey, sugar, bay leaves, butter and bread crumbs" (Braudel, 1967, p. 167).

6. Although some suggest that it was the Chinese who discovered distillation (e.g., Hyams, 1965, p. 226), others believe it was the Italians (e.g., Braudel, 1967, p. 170) and some name the Greeks (e.g., Forbes, 1948, p. 6), most assert that it was the Arabians (e.g., Patrick, 1952, p. 29; Lichine, 1974, p. 6). But if it was indeed the Arabians, was it the physician Rhazer (852?-932?) (Waddell & Haag, 1940, p. 58) or the alchemist Jabir in Hayyan around 800 A.D. (Roueché, 1963, p. 171)? Perhaps it was all of the above: "That spirit could be distilled from fermented matter was undoubtedly independently discovered (possibly by accident) in many parts of the world" (Doxat, 1971, p. 80). It might be noted parenthetically that alcohol (*al kohl* or *alkuhl*) is Arabic in name (Hyams, 1965, p. 198; Roueché, 1963, p. 171).

7. Arnaldus of Villanova (d. 1315), a professor of medicine, is credited with coining the term *aqua vitae*: "We call it [distilled liquor] aqua vitae, and this name is remarkably suitable, since it is really a water of immortality. It prolongs life, clears away ill-humors, revives the heart, and maintains youth" (Arnaldus de Villanova, *The Earliest Printed Book on Wine, Now for the First Time Rendered into English, and with an Historical Essay by H.E. Sigerist, with Facsimile of Original Edition, 1478.* New York: Schuman's, 1943, cited by Roueché, 1963, p. 172). These were modest claims compared to those made much later by the fifteenth-century German physician, Hieronymus Brunschwig:

> It eases the diseases coming of cold. It comforts the heart. It heals all old and new sores on the head. It causes a good color in a person. It heals baldness and causes the hair well to grow, and kills lice and fleas. It cures lethargy. Cotton wet in the same time and a little wrung out again and so put in the ears at night going to bed, and a little drunk thereof, is of good against all deafness. It eases the pain in the teeth, and causes sweet breath. It heals the canker in the mouth, in the teeth, in the lips, and in the tongue. It causes the heavy tongue to become light and well-speaking. It heals the short breath. It causes good digestion and appetite for to eat, and takes away all belching. It draws the wind out of the body. It eases the yellow jaundice, the dropsy, the gout, the pain in the breasts when they be swollen, and heals all diseases in the bladder, and breaks the stone. It withdraws venom that has been taken in meat or in drink, when a little treacle is put thereto. It heals all shrunken sinews, and causes them to become soft and right. It heals the fevers tertian and quartan. It heals the bites of a mad dog, and all stinking wounds, when they be washed therewith. It gives also young courage in a person, and causes him to have a good memory. It purifies the five wits of melancholy and of all uncleanness." (H. Brunschwig, *Liber de Arte Distillandi: De Simplicibus*, Strasbourg, 1500, quoted by Roueché, 1963, pp. 172-173).

8. The Russians preferred their grain spirit without the juniper flavor, and chose to name it "vodka," or "little water" (Roueché, 1963, p. 174).

9. Alarmist tracts exaggerated the extent of problems and "the popular press was full of terrifying accounts of the woes of prostitution and infanticide . . ." (Sournia, 1990, p. 21). An influential engraving by William Hogarth pictures a society destroyed by gin. Life on "Gin Lane" is portrayed a living hell in which, among other things, an intoxicated mother neglects her child, who is seen falling on its head, and an impoverished man gnaws on the end of a bone (bearing a suspicious resemblance to a human femur) while a hungry dog chews at the other end. A drunken brawl can be seen in the background and a dead woman, who presumably succumbed to gin, is being placed in a coffin. "Gin

Lane" has been reproduced in numerous publications, including Sournia (1990, illustration #9), Babor (1986, p. 18), Watney (1974, illustration #2), Watney (1976, illustration #1), and Younger (1966, p. 334).

10.   The Act attempted to create a de facto prohibition, especially among the poor, but was far from successful:

> As was proved in the U.S.A. in our own times, try to prohibit liquor and you end by encouraging it. The fact that gin was largely illegal made it the more attractive and undoubtedly this fact alone caused some who would not otherwise have touched it to be tempted to try it and possibly thus to become addicted to it. Illicit gin shops flourished, and though some 12,000 persons were found guilty, it was difficult to enforce fines: the prisons were too crowded anyway. Informers, who alone could provide evidence, tended to suffer mysterious and often fatal accidents. The law was brought into contempt, always a bad thing (Doxat, 1972, pp. 99-100).

11.   To the pre-Christian Anglo-Saxons, heaven was not a place to play harps but a place to visit with other departed and drink plentiful and endless draughts of delicious ale (Watney, 1974, p. 15).

REFERENCES

Alcoholism and Drug Addiction Research Foundation of Ontario. "It's Best to Know" About Alcoholism. Toronto, Ontario: Alcoholism and Drug Addiction Research Foundation of Ontario, 1961.

Alcoholism and Drug Addiction Research Foundation of Ontario (booklet), 1961.

Ashton, Thomas S. *An Economic History of England: The Eighteenth Century.* London: Methuen and Co., 1955.

Austin, Gregory A. *Alcohol in Western Society from Antiquity to 1800: A Chronological History.* Santa Barbara, CA: ABC - Clio, 1985.

Babor, Thomas. Alcohol: Customs and Rituals. New York: Chelsea House, 1986.

Balazs, Etienne. *Chinese Civilization and Bureaucracy.* New Haven, CT: Yale University Press, 1964. (Translated by H. M. Wright).

Baron, Stanley. *Brewed in America: A History of Beer and Ale in the United States.* Boston: Little, Brown and Co., 1962.

Blacker, Edward. Sociocultural factors in alcoholism. *International Psychiatry Clinics*, 1966, *3*, 51-80.

Blum, Richard H., and Associates. *Society and Drugs.* San Francisco, CA: Jossey Bass, 1969.

Boffeta, Paolo, and Garfinkel, Lawrence. Alcohol drinking and mortality among men enrolled in an American Cancer Society prospective study. *Epidemiology*, 1990, *1*, 342-348.

Braidwood, Robert J., Sauer, Jonathan D., Helbaek, Hans, Mangelsdorf, Paul C., Cutler,

Hugh C., Coon, Careton S., Linton, Ralph, Steward, Julian, and Oppenheim, A. Leo. Symposium: Did man once live by beer alone? *American Anthropologist*, 1953, *55*, 515-526.

Braudel, Fernand. *Capitalism and Material Life, 1400-1800*. Translated by Miriam Kochan. New York, NY: Harper and Row, 1974.

Chafetz, Morris E. *Liquor: The Servant of Man*. Boston: Little, Brown and Co., 1965.

Cherrington, Ernest H. (ed.) *Standard Encyclopedia of the Alcohol Problem*. 6 vols. Westerville, OH: American Issue Publishing Co., 1925-1930.

Claudian, J. History of the Usage of Alcohol. In: Tremoiliers, J. (ed.) *International Encyclopedia of Pharmacology and Therapeutics*. Section 20, vol. 1. Oxford: Pergamon, 1970. pp. 3-26.

Darby, William J., Ghaliounqui, Paul, and Grivetti, Louis. *Food: The Gift of Osiris*. Vols. 1 and 2. London: Academic Press, 1977.

DeLabry, Lorraine O., Glynn, Robert J., Levenson, Michael R., Hermos, John A., LoCastro, Joseph S, and Vokonas, Pantel S. Alcohol consumption and mortality in an American male population: Recovering the U-shape curve-findings from the Normative Aging Study. *Journal of Studies on Alcohol*, 1992, *53*, 25-32.

Doxat, John. *The World of Drinks and Drinking*. New York: Drake Publishers, 1971.

Fei-Peng, Zhang. Drinking in China. *The Drinking and Drug Practice Surveyor*, 1982, No. 18, 12-15.

Forbes, R. J. *Short History of the Art of Distillation*. Leiden: E. J. Brill, 1948.

French, Henry V. *Nineteen Centuries of Drink in England: A History*. 2nd. edition London: National Temperance Publication Depot, 1890.

Gastineau, Clifford F., Darby, William J., and Turner, Thomas B. (eds.) *Fermented Foods in Nutrition*. New York: Academic Press, 1979.

Gavaler, Judith S. and Van Thiel, David H. The association between moderate alcoholic beverage consumption and serum estradiol and testosterone levels in normal post menopausal women: relationship to the literature. *Alcohol: Clinical and Experimental Research*, 1992, 16, 87-92.

Gernet, Jacques. *Daily Life in China on the Eve of the Mongol Invasion 1250-1276*. Stanford, CA: Stanford University Press, 1962. (Translated by H. M. Wright).

Ghaliounqui, Paul. Fermented Beverages in Antiquity. In: Gastineau, Clifford F., Darby, William J., and Turner, Thomas B. (eds.) *Fermented Food Beverages in Nutrition*. New York: Academic Press, 1979. pp. 3-19.

Granet, Marcel. *Chinese Civilization*. London: Barnes and Noble, 1957.

Hewitt, T. Furman. *A Biblical Perspective on the Use and Abuse of Alcohol and Other Drugs*. Raleigh, NC: North Carolina Department of Human Resources, Pastoral Care Council on Alcohol and Drug Abuse, 1980.

Hucker, Charles O. *China's Imperial Past*. Stanford, CA: Stanford University Press, 1975.

Hyams, Edward. *Dionysus: A Social History of the Wine Vine*. New York: Macmillan, 1965.

Jackson, Rodney, Scargg, Robert, and Beaglehole, Robert. Alcohol consumption and risk of coronary heart disease. *British Medical Journal*, 1991, 303, 211-215.

Jellinek, E. Morton. Drinkers and Alcoholics in Ancient Rome. *Journal of Studies on Alcohol*, 37: 1718-1741, 1976.

Katz, S. H. and Voigt, M. M. Bread and beer: The early use of cereals in the human diet. *Expedition*, 1987, *28*, 23-34.

Keller, Mark. The great Jewish drink mystery. *British Journal of Addiction*, 1970, *64*, 287-296.

King, Frank A. *Beer Has a History*. London: Hutchinson's Scientific and Technical Publications, 1947.

Klatsky, Arthur L., Armstrong, Mary Anne, and Friedman, Gary D. Risk of cardiovascular mortality in alcohol drinkers, ex-drinkers and nondrinkers. *The American Journal of Cardiology*, 1990, *66*, 1237-1242.

Lausanne, Edita. *The Great Book of Wine*. New York: World Publishing Co., 1969.

Lazar, Irving, and Ford, John. Untitled reaction of review panel. In: Lauderdale, Michael L. *An Analysis of the Control Theory of Alcoholism*. Denver, CO: Education Commission of the States, 1977. pp. 29-34.

Lichine, Alexis. *Alexis Lichine's New Encyclopedia of Wines and Spirits*. 2nd. edition. New York: Knopf, 1974.

Lucia, Salvatore P. *A History of Wine as Therapy*. Philadelphia, PA: J. B. Lippincott, 1963a.

Lucia, Salvatore P. The Antiquity of Alcohol in Diet and Medicine. In: Lucia, Salvatore P. (ed.) *Alcohol and Civilization*. New York: McGraw-Hill, 1963b. pp. 151-166.

Lutz, H. F. *Viticulture and Brewing in the Ancient Orient*. New York: J. C. Heinrichs, 1922.

Magee, Malachy. *1000 Years of Irish Whiskey*. Dublin, Ireland: O'Brien Press, 1980.

Marciniak, Marek L. Filters, Strainers and Siphons in Wine and Beer Production and Drinking Customs in Ancient Egypt. Paper presented at Annual Alcohol Epidemiology Symposium of the Kettil Bruun Society for Social and Epidemiological Research on Alcohol. Toronto, Ontario: May 30-June 5, 1992.

Mathias, Peter. *The Brewing Industry in England, 1700 - 1830*. Cambridge: Cambridge University Press, 1959.

Miller, G. J., Beckles, G. L. A., Maude, G. H., and Carson, D. C. Alcohol consumption: Protection against coronary heart disease and risks to health. *International Journal of Epidemiology*, 1990, *19*, 923-930.

Monckton, Herbert A. *A History of English Ale and Beer*. London: Bodley Head, 1966.

O'Brien, John M., and Seller, Sheldon C. Attributes of Alcohol in the Old Testament. *The Drinking and Drug Practices Surveyor*, 1982, No. 18, 18-24.

Patai, Raphael. From "Journey Into the Jewish Mind" - Alcoholism. In: Blaine, Allan (ed.) *Alcoholism and the Jewish Community*. New York: Commission on Synagogue Relations, Federation of Jewish Philanthropies of New York, 1980. pp. 61-87.

Patrick, Charles H. *Alcohol, Culture, and Society*. Durham, NC: Duke University Press, 1952. Reprint edition by AMS Press, New York, 1970.

Popham, Robert E. The Social History of the Tavern. In: Israel, Yedy, Glaser, Frederick B., Kalant, Harold, Popham, Robert E., Schmidt, Wolfgang, and Smart, Reginald G. (eds.) *Research Advances in Alcohol and Drug Problems*. Vol. 4. New York: Plenum Press, 1978. pp. 225-302.

Porter, Roy. Introduction. In: Sournia, Jean-Charles. *A History of Alcoholism*. Trans. by Nick Hindley and Gareth Stanton. Oxford: Basil Blackwell, 1990. pp. ix-xvi.

Raymond, Irving W. *The Teaching of the Early Church on the Use of Wine and Strong Drink*. New York: Columbia University Press, 1927.

Razay, G., Heaton, K. W., Bolton, C. H., and Hughes, A. O. Alcohol consumption and its relation to cardiovascular risk factors in British women. *British Medical Journal*, 1992, *304*, 80-83.

Rimm, Eric B., Giovannucci, Edward L., Willett, Walter C., Colditz, Graham A., Ascherio, Alberto, Rosner, Bernard, and Stampfer, Meir J. Prospective study of alcohol consumption and risk of coronary heart disease in men. *The Lancet*, 1991, *338*, 464-468.

Rorabaugh, William J. *The Alcoholic Republic: An American Tradition*. New York, NY: Oxford University Press, 1979.

Roueché, Berton. *The Neutral Spirit: A Portrait of Alcohol*. Boston: Little, Brown and Co., 1960.

Roueché, Berton. Alcohol in Human Culture. In: Lucia, Salvatore P. (ed.) *Alcohol and Civilization*. New York: McGraw-Hill, 1963. pp. 167-182.

Royce, James E. Sin or Solace? Religious Views on Alcohol and Alcoholism. In: Watts, Thomas D. (ed.) *Social Thought on Alcoholism: A Comprehensive Review*. Malabar, FL: Robert E. Krieger Publishing Co., 1986. pp. 53-66.

Samuelson, James. *The History of Drink*. London: Trubner and Co., 1878.

Seward, Desmond. *Monks and Wine*. London: Mitchell Beazley Publishers, 1979.

Simoons, Frederick J. *Food in China: A Cultural and Historical Inquiry*. Boca Raton, FL: CRC Press, 1991.

Slavin, Arthur J. *The Way of the West: The Reorganization of Europe, 1300-1760*. Vol. 2. Lexington, MA: Xerox College Publishing, 1973.

Sournia, Jean-Charles. *A History of Alcoholism*. Trans. by Nick Hindley and Gareth Stanton. Oxford: Basil Blackwell, 1990.

Spiegel, Marcia C. The Heritage of Noah: Alcoholism in the Jewish Community Today. Unpublished M.A. thesis, Hebrew Union College-Jewish Institute of Religion, 1979.

Steinkraus, Keith H. Nutritionally Significant Indigenous Foods Involving an Alcoholic Fermentation. In: Gastineau, Clifford F., Darby, William J., and Turner, Thomas B. (eds.) *Fermented Food Beverages in Nutrition*. New York: Academic Press, 1979. pp. 35-57.

Waddell, James A., and Haag, H. B. *Alcohol in Moderation and Excess*. Richmond, VA: 1940.

Wallbank, T. Walter, and Taylor, Alastair M. *Civilization: Past and Present*. Vol. 1. 3rd edition. Chicago, IL: Scott, Foresman and Co., 1954.

Watney, John. *Mother's Ruin: A History of Gin*. London: Peter Owen, 1976.

Watney, John. *Beer is Best: A History of Beer*. London: Peter Owen, 1974.

Wilson, C. Anne. *Food and Drink in Britain from the Stone Age to the 19th Century*. Chicago: Academy Chicago Publishers, 1991.

Wilson, John. *Scotland's Malt Whiskies*. Alexandria, VA: Famedram Publishers, 1973.

Younger, William A. *Gods, Men, and Wine*. London: Wine and Food Society; Michael Joseph, 1966.

2

Alcohol Around the World

Most societies and groups around the world use alcohol and experience few problems because cultural expectations heavily influence how alcohol affects those who consume it. It does not physiologically "disinhibit" the brain; intoxicated behavior conforms to cultural expectations. Such behavior is virtually always within the limits seen by the society as acceptable for the circumstances. Drinking problems are minimized when drinking is considered normal behavior; is a reflection and expression of social relationships, religious practices, and customs learned early at home; is an activity often occurring with meals; and when drinking behaviors are regulated and controlled by custom in a widely-known and accepted manner (Robbins, 1979, p. 363).

PRELITERATE GROUPS

Alcohol Use Varies Widely Around World

While the substance of ethanol is invariant throughout the world, societal reaction to it ranges from total rejection to "avid immersion" (Mandelbaum, 1979, p. 14). For example, among the Kofyar of northern Nigeria, life revolves around making and drinking beer (Netting, 1979), and among the Tarahumara of Mexico, the most important and consistent pattern of interpersonal relationship beyond those within the household occurs within the context of the tesgüinada, or beer drinking party. That cultural institution is "*the major structural form* of the Tarahumara social system above the family and residence group" (Kennedy, 1978, pp. 125-126, emphasis in original) and is desirable and highly functional for their society. Among the Abipone of Paraguay, those who abstain from alcohol are thought to be "cowardly, degenerate and stupid" (Dobrizhoffer, 1822, p. 432, cited by Washburne, 1961, p. 86).

While most societies consider alcohol to be valuable, a few view it as destructive and undesirable. For example, the Hopi and other Pueblo peoples of the Southwestern United States (for whom alcohol was not known before Columbus) believed that drinking alcohol threatened their way of life. They abhorred the use of alcohol so strongly that they successfully banned it from their communities for many years (Mandelbaum, 1979).

Alcohol is often perceived very differently around the world. To some it is a food, while to others it is a poison; to some it is a tranquilizer, while to others it is an aphrodisiac; to some it is a sacred substance or a way to know God, while to others it is sacrilegious and paves the way to eternal damnation. In some societies drunkenness is valued as a religious experience, while in others it is rejected or disgusting; in some it is a crime, while in others it absolves or reduces responsibility for one's behavior; in some it is welcomed as a social lubricant, while in others it is rejected as a threat to proper social interaction (Heath, 1987, pp. 24-25).[1]

It is important to view the use of alcohol as culturally defined and socially structured:

Drinking behavior in a particular society is viewed most adequately within the context of a way of life. Though certain concentrations of ingested alcohol have consistent physiological effects on the human organism, the effects of drinking on behavior vary in important aspects from society to society. For example, the use of alcohol may, but does not necessarily, result in heightened aggression and sexuality. Drinking, even when "excessive," is typically social behavior subject to group control. Who will drink what, when, where and with whom are rarely, if ever, matters of chance alone. Moreover, drinking which results repeatedly in getting drunk does not necessarily result in alcoholism, and the association of sin and guilt with all drinking is apparently confined largely to segments of modern western society (Maddox and McCall, 1964, p. 19).

"Norms and cultural expectations affect not only how people react to the idea of alcohol and to people who use it, but also heavily influence how it affects those who consume it" (Bacon and Jones, 1968, p. 12; MacAndrew and Edgerton, 1969). As one anthropologist (Mandelbaum, 1979, p. 15)[2] stresses that

. . . the behavioral consequences of drinking alcohol depends as much on a people's idea of what alcohol does to a person as they do on the physiological processes that take place [cf. Washburne 1961]. When a man lifts a cup, it is not only the kind of drink that is in it, the amount he is likely to take, and the circumstances under which he will do the drinking that are specified in advance for him, but also whether the contents of the cup will cheer or stupefy, whether they will induce affection or aggression, guilt or unalloyed pleasure. These and many other cultural definitions attach to the drink even before it touches the lips.

"In most societies, drinking is essentially a social act and, as such, it is embedded in a context of values, attitudes, and other norms. These values, attitudes, and other norms constitute important socio-cultural factors that influence the effects of drinking, regardless of how important biochemical, physiological, and pharmacokinetic factors may also be in that respect" (Heath, 1987, p. 46).

This very important point has been documented by many, but none better than by MacAndrew and Edgerton (1969) in their classic *Drunken Comportment: A Social Explanation.* The authors demonstrate the inadequacy of the commonly held belief that alcohol acts upon the "higher center of the brain" as a "moral incapacitator" to account for the wide diversity of behavior that occurs under intoxication both within and between societies around the world. "What we actually find when we examine the phenomenon of drunkenness as it occurs throughout the world is a series of infinite gradations in the degree of 'disinhibition' that is manifested in drunken comportment" (MacAndrew and Edgerton, 1969, p. 17).

People in Many Societies Do Not Become Disinhibited When Intoxicated

The Yuruna are a fierce, head-hunting people in the Xingú River region of the South American tropical forest. While they consume substantial quantities of *malicha* (made from fermented manioc root), they do not become disinhibited but rather withdraw entirely into themselves and behave much as though no one else existed (Nimuendajú, 1948, p. 238 cited by MacAndrew and Edgerton, 1969, p. 17).

Similarly, the residents of Vicos in the Peruvian Andes have engaged in ceremonial drinking since pre-Columbian days, and drinking remains "an integral feature of both formal and informal community life" (MacAndrew and Edgerton, 1969, p. 17). Presently,

[i]n Vicos, small children are given corn beer and everyone over 16 years of age drinks (aguardiente). Drinking by most adults, particularly adult males, is usually followed by drunkenness, and in many instances a man or woman may be drunk for several days in succession. The incidence and frequency of drinking and the amounts consumed seem to be very high. Drinking is a social activity, however, and drinking customs are integrated with the most basic and powerful institutions in the community. Drinking and drunkenness do not seem to lead to any breakdown in interpersonal relations, nor do they seem to interfere with the performance of social roles by individuals (Mangin, 1957, p. 58, cited in MacAndrew and Edgerton, 1969, p. 18).

Mangin views the role of alcohol for the Vicosino to be "prevailingly integrative." He further notes:

Sexual activity of a premarital variety appears to increase during fiestas, but this may not be a function of drinking. Several male informants told the author that they purposely stayed sober at times during fiestas so that they could "escape" with a girl. Extramarital sexual activity, which is a disruptive force in Vicos culture, seems to occur mostly when individuals are quite sober. . . . Most of the crimes committed by Vicosinos during the field study were carried out while sober. In only two cases (one of which occurred before the [21 month] field study and one during it) could be documented that drunkenness was associated with criminality (Mangin, 1957, p. 63, cited in MacAndrew and Edgerton, 1969, p. 18).

The Camba of Eastern Bolivia live in an isolated section of the country, and their way of life has changed little since the Spanish colonial period. They drink, undiluted, a distillate of cane sugar which is 89% ethyl alcohol and which they appropriately call *alcohol*. "The behavioral patterns associated with drinking are so formalized as to constitute a secular ritual" and "are the only way in which the Camba drink, except at wakes where a different but equally formalized pattern of behavior is followed" (Heath, 1958, pp. 499-500).

Ritualized, extended drinking parties usually begin shortly after breakfast, and drinkers (men, women, and children as young as 12) consume *alcohol* until they fall asleep or pass out. Upon awakening, consumption resumes until the drinkers again pass out. This cycle is repeated, day and night until all the *alcohol* is consumed or until they must return to work (Heath, 1958, pp. 500-501, cited in MacAndrew and Edgerton, pp. 20-21). Thus intoxication is normative; it is sought, expected and supported by the group. Nevertheless, there is no evidence whatsoever of individual dependence on alcohol nor of disinhibition of any kind (physical or verbal) associated with intoxication (Heath, 1962, pp. 25-26 and 30).

Heath suggests that " . . . alcohol plays a predominantly integrative role in Camba society, where drinking is an elaborately ritualized group activity and alcoholism is unknown. The anxieties which are often cited as bases for common group drinking are not present, but fiestas constitute virtually the only corporate form of social expression. Drinking parties predominate among rare social activities, and alcohol serves to facilitate rapport between individuals who are normally isolated and introverted" (Heath, 1962, p. 35).

Another society in which disinhibition does not occur during drunkenness is illustrated by the Mestizo village of Aritama in northern Columbia. The Aritama are inordinately self-conscious and wear a rigid mask of seriousness beneath which is a high level of hostility. This hostility even extends to relations between spouses, between parents and their children, between generations and between siblings.

Regardless of the occasion and the degree of intoxication, the Aritama maintain their "rigid mask of seriousness." The Reichel-Dolmatoffs report, "There is never open physical aggressiveness of serious proportions, nor is there merry socializing, romantic serenading, obscene talk, or political discussion of any kind. One man will sing, perhaps, another play the drum or rattle, while the others sit and listen, drinking in silence and only rarely making physical contacts or attempts at conversation" (Reichel-Dolmatoff, 1961, p. 197, cited by MacAndrew and Edgerton, 1969, pp. 24-25). Elsewhere they write, "A man might drink and drum all night long without once losing his composure, without becoming aggressive, sentimental, verbose, or amorous" (1961, p. 113, cited by MacAndrew and Edgerton, 1969, p. 25).

A similar lack of disinhibition while intoxicated is found among the inhabitants of the small atoll of Ifaluk in the Caroline Islands of the South Pacific. In this society there are no overt expressions of hostility among adults. However, the resulting harmony is at the expense of dogs, who are viciously mistreated scapegoats. Does alcohol disinhibit drinkers and release their pent-up hostility, leading to verbal and physical attacks? Not at all. The anthropologists Burrows and Spiro reported "Some of the men drink glass after glass in the course of an evening. A slightly bleary look about the eyes, and a tendency to be jovial or sentimentally friendly, were the only effects we noticed" (Burrows and Spiro, 1953, p. 44, cited by MacAndrew and Edgerton, 1969, p. 28). Burrows wrote that "indulgence in coconut toddy[3] seemed to have a mellowing effect. We never saw or heard of a 'fighting drunk'" (Burrows, 1952, p. 24, cited by MacAndrew and Edgerton, 1969, p. 28). These descriptions of intoxicated behavior among the Ifaluk are corroborated by the independent observations of others (Bates and Abbott, 1958).

Intoxication also fails to produce disinhibited behavior among residents on the fishing island of Takashima off the coast of Japan in the Inland Sea. Aggression is suppressed, as are expressions of sexuality, obscenity and discussion of anything sexual in nature. An anthropologist (Norbeck, 1954, pp. 87-88, 155) has reported that they become friendly, happy and jovial when intoxicated (and many become *highly* intoxicated); they do *not* become aggressive or sexual in speech or act. In his words, "Continued drinking soon leads to a good-natured drunkenness, camaraderie, laughter, jokes, songs and dances, which are considered the inevitable result if not the objective of continued drinking" (Norbeck, 1954, p. 72, cited in MacAndrew and Edgerton, 1969, p. 33).

Yet another society in which intoxication might be expected to lead to "disinhibited" behavior, but does not, is that of the Mixtec people of Juxtlahuaca in the state of Oaxaca, Mexico. The Mixtecans value tranquility and suppress jealousy, anger, and aggression, emotions which they believe lead to illness; consequently they are rarely if ever overtly aggressive when sober. Anthropologists report that the Mixtecans "specifically deny" that alcohol can produce aggression in them. They also report having repeatedly observed Mixtecans drink themselves into high levels of intoxication but never having observed them become loud or aggressive (Romney and Romney, 1963, p. 611).

Intoxicated Behavior Conforms to Social Norms

MacAndrew and Edgerton have convincingly demonstrated that alcohol does not act upon the brain in some way so as to bring about "moral disinhibition." But why does such disinhibition appear to occur in some societies? Chandler

Washburne (1961, p. 258) observed that ". . . the kinds of behavior we will observe when people are drinking depend upon the personality changes and the cultural norms surrounding alcohol, and the occasions on which it is used." He was interested in the expression of aggression when persons are intoxicated and noted, "In one society after another it can be seen that aggression is highly patterned, indicative of the norms governing behavior (Washburne, 1961, p. 261).

Washburne also observed that the objects of aggression are limited by a society's norms. In some societies, like the Cuna of Central America, women are never subject to aggression by intoxicated men. In others, like the Ainu of northern Japan and some African groups, men are likely to assault their wives when drunk (Washburne, 1961, p. 262). Spousal assault (perpetrated both by husband and wives) is common in our society, but physical assault upon parents is not common.[4] Among the Chamula of the Central American highlands, who are well-known for their violence when intoxicated, children are never the objects of violence (Bunzel, 1940, p. 377).

It was Washburne's (1961, p. 262) belief that when people begin to drink they have a series of expectations about their drinking behavior and that their behavior while intoxicated will follow the patterns established by society. Therefore, the most strongly prohibited forms of aggression are not likely to occur no matter how intoxicated people become; what usually occurs are the socially tolerated forms. He observed that "There are wide differences, even among groups in the United States, in regard to the amount of physical aggression permitted when drinking, and the typical behavior of members does not exceed the tolerated limit beyond which sanctions begin to be involved" (Washburne, 1961, p. 262).

Drinking Behavior Stays "Within the Limits"

MacAndrew and Edgerton (1969, p. 67) believe that a "within-the-limits clause" governs drunken excesses. By that term they "refer to the fact that, with rare exceptions, for even the most seemingly disinhibited drunkard there are limits beyond which he does not go." Marshall (1979, p. 453) concludes, "All societies recognize permissible alterations in behavior from normal, sober comportment when alcoholic beverages are consumed, but these alterations are always 'within limits.'" He also notes that these limits are more lax than those for sober persons in the same situations.

An example of the "within-the-limits" clause is found among the Thonga of South Africa, who enjoy a long drinking carnival (the luma festival) lasting at least several weeks. The Thonga say that at the luma festival "the law is no longer in force" (Junod, 1927, p. 402, cited by Washburne, 1961, p. 48), an assertion which Washburne qualifies, "Many ordinary rules of conduct may be violated, but in a sense they are not violated because they do not apply in this situation. One's role in society is changed as a participant in the festival, and new social expectations replace the old. That this is a social invention and not merely the result of alcohol releasing inhibitions can be seen by the fact that often duties, such as the passing of taxes to the chief, go on at this time" (Washburne, 1961, p. 48).

In the words of another observer, "How far does sexual license go at the time of the bukanye (luma)? Not to the point of general promiscuity . . . however, many cases of adultery occur" (Junod, 1927, p. 402, quoted in Washburne, 1961, p. 49). In other words, the behavior operates within the limits set by society for the luma festival.

The Siriono of southeastern Bolivia do most of their drinking in what might be called parties or bouts. Quarreling is a part of everyday life and aggression commonly occurs during drinking episodes. Washburne (1961, pp. 118-119) explains that

. . . although the drinking bout offers a chance to discharge aggression and bring up problems of sex or food that one is disturbed about, the situation is still controlled by social norms. When drinking, the inhibitions are not simply removed, leaving the individual free to discharge his aggression as he will. There are socially approved methods, and these norms regulate behavior when aggressive acts take place. Thus aggression when drinking is not a case of ignoring or violating the rules of the society. It is expected and permitted, but only within the well-defined rules and regulations of quarreling and fighting. This cannot be looked upon as unsocialized behavior. There is a tendency to think that the aggression that may follow heavy drinking occurs because the individual is no longer able to remember the rules of social conduct and govern his behavior by them. Among the Siriono there is certainly an increase in overt aggression, but the individuals are still following rules laid down by their society to govern aggressive behavior.

The cannibalistic Tupinamba of Brazil drink to reach a high level of intoxication, during which they are able to engage in extreme behavior. Their sober behavior tends to be characterized by laughing, joking and sociability. Their intoxicated behavior is generally consistent with their sober behavior, being only more intensified. "A kind a role change is seen in the comic part one can play when drinking, in that silly and antic behavior is admired, rewarded and encouraged, apparently in special patterned forms" (Washburne, 1961, p. 132). Thus, the extreme intoxicated behavior appears to conform to social expectations.

Among the Cuna of Panama and Columbia, men and women become intoxicated for several days at a time (Stout, 1947, pp. 94-95; Wafer, 1934, p. 100; both cited in Washburne, 1961, p. 148). It appears that "there is a status assigned to a person when drunk, with certain expected and prohibited types of behavior" (Washburne, 1961, p. 148). Thus, intoxicated persons play or enact a socially defined role which permits certain behaviors and prohibits others. While drunken festivals "are often a source of fights, defiance of cultural mores, and so forth," there are clearly specified limits to such aggression. For example, "No instance is known, or recorded in literature, of a Cuna man quarreling with or abusing his wife, even while drunk" (Marshall, 1950, pp. 338, 343-344, cited in Washburne, 1961, p. 149). Similarly, there is no breakdown of norms regarding sexual behavior. Thus, behavior rules appear to govern intoxicated behavior effectively.

The Lepchas of the Himalayas are preoccupied with sex and are, by almost anyone's standards, inordinately promiscuous. "Sex is, indeed, almost the people's sole recreation, and the most common topic of conversation on practically every occasion" (Morris, 1938, p. 220, cited by MacAndrew and Edgerton, 1969, p. 79). During the annual harvest festival there is much drinking and dancing throughout the day. Anyone who dances must spend the night in the fields, where the ordinary rules of conduct are relaxed and the more copulating couples the better. "On that night anybody may sleep with anyone else provided the rules of incest are not broken" (Gorer, 1938, p. 242, cited in MacAndrew and Edgerton, 1969, p. 81). This is easier said than done, because the Lepchas have a highly complex definition of incest which includes blood relations for nine generations on the father's side and four on the mother's, plus numerous relations by marriage. Yet no matter how intoxicated they become, the Lepchas do not violate the taboo (MacAndrew and Edgerton, 1969, pp. 80-81).

Acceptable Behavior Varies According to Situation

Importantly, the norms guiding drinking (including intoxicated behavior) vary according to the situation. For example, among the Maori of North Island, New Zealand, the consumption of alcohol occurs in either drinking "sessions" or drinking "parties." At drinking sessions, people tend to become drowsy and relaxed. However, at drinking parties, they tend to become "gay and noisy." Behavior in the two situations is also different. "In the later stages of parties, violence is quite common (out of six parties held in one weekend four finished with a fight). There is also a sexual undertone at parties which is quite absent from sessions" (Ritchie, 1963, p. 80).

When men and women drink together among the Taira of Okinawa, drunken aggression never occurs. However, when men drink by themselves, it does. Similarly, when the Tecospans of Mexico drink among themselves, violence never occurs. But when they drink with outsiders, they often become involved in disputes, conflict and fighting (MacAndrew and Edgerton, 1969, pp. 55-57).

There are two very different ways the Chichicastenango of Guatemala conduct themselves when intoxicated. When they drink ceremonially, as they did long before contact with Europeans, men retain their dignity and fulfill their ceremonial duties. And they do this even when they become so intoxicated they are unable to walk. However, when they drink in bars and taverns where secular and European culture controls the situation, they dance, quarrel and become sexually promiscuous (Bunzel, 1940, p. 367).

The Chippewa of Minnesota exhibit two drinking styles that Westermeyer (1972) labels "white drinking" and "Indian drinking." The former is characterized by restraint and drinkers act much as they do when not drinking. The latter is characterized by heightened emotions, such as euphoria, depression, joy and anger. Arguments, fights and suicide attempts are common. Most Chippewa drink white style on occasion. However, "One can observe the same person drinking in this manner at a white bar, and in the same evening observe him drinking 'Indian style' at an Indian bar. Chippewa acquaintances, unexpectedly meeting the author in an Indian bar, have dropped Indian drinking behavior and assumed white drinking for the course of the conversation" (Westermeyer, 1972, p. 400).

Among the men of Truk in Micronesia, drinking results in radically different ways over their life cycle. Their conduct while intoxicated varies according to their age and to social expectations about appropriate behavior for men of that age. Young men are expected to be brave and therefore tend to engage in brawls and other acts of bravado. By their mid-thirties they relinquish this "young man" role and are expected to be responsible "mature men." While they drink as much as the young men, they subject themselves to public ridicule if they conduct themselves as their younger compatriots do. "The same beverages are consumed by the same person in approximately the same amounts at different times in their lives. . . . Their inhibitions do not tighten up with advancing years. What has changed is the set of public expectations surrounding appropriate behavior for men at different stations in life" (Marshall, 1979a, p. 116).

In Colonial Mexico, drunken violence rarely occurred in central Mexico and Oaxaca during community feasts, harvest rites and other group rituals that reinforced community bonds. However, it did occur much more often in unstructured situations in which drinking did not signify social responsibility (Taylor, 1979, p. 66).

The "within-the-limits" phenomenon has been described among such North American groups as the Navajo (Levy and Kunitz, 1974, p. 187), the Teton Sioux (Mohatt, 1972, p. 266), the Yankton Sious (Hurt and Brown, 1965, p. 229), the Potawatoni (Hamer, 1980, p. 118), the Cree (Kupferer, 1979, p. 202), the Aleuts (Berreman, 1956, pp. 507-508), and the Hare (Savishinsky, 1977, p. 46).

It has also been described elsewhere among the Etal people of Micronesia (Nason, 1979, p. 247), the Admiralty Islanders of northwestern Melanesia (Schwartz and Romanucci-Ross, 1979, pp. 258-265), the Japanese (Yamamuro, 1979, p. 277; Sargent, 1979, pp. 279-280), the Bantu of South Africa (Hutchinson, 1979, p. 329), the Kofyar of West Africa (Netting, 1979, p. 359), the Baganda of Uganda (Robbins, 1979, p. 369), German-speaking Austrian villagers of Central Europe (Honigmann, 1979, pp. 427-428), the Dusun of North Borneo (Washburne, 1961, pp. 248-249), the Yakut of northeastern Siberia (Washburne, 1961, pp. 234 and 239), the Tarahumara of northern Mexico (Washburne, 1961, p. 162), the Kaingáng of Brazil (Henry, 1941, pp. 62-63), the Abipone of Paraguay (Dobrizhoffer, 1822, v. 2, p. 66) and the Pondo of South Africa (Hunter, 1961, pp. 369-370), among others.

Genetics Can not Explain Differences in Behaviors

Genetic differences would appear inadequate to explain such differences in behavior. For example, the Ifaluk conduct themselves very differently than do their neighbors on nearby atolls, who have the same biological or genetic "stock." Nor can genetic differences explain dramatic and widespread variation in drunken comportment from situation to situation. This led MacAndrew and Edgerton to conclude:

Since the ingestion of alcohol is sometimes followed by the most flagrant imaginable changes in comportment, sometimes by only moderate changes, and sometimes by no significant changes whatsoever, it seems evident that *in and of itself, the presence of alcohol in the body does not necessarily even conduce to disinhibition, much less inevitably produce such an effect.* This is not to say, however, that what one does when he is drunk is a merely capricious affair, for once the socially organized character of drunken comportment is recognized, the notion that it is guided by nothing more substantial than the impulse of the moment can no longer be sustained. And since no one would seriously entertain, much less defend, the possibility that persons are born in possession of all manner of fine distinctions as to what properly goes with what-- distinctions that are selectively exercised during drunkenness--we must conclude that drunken comportment is an essentially *learned* affair (1969, pp. 87-88, emphasis in original).

They explain, that *"Over the course of socialization, people learn about drunkenness what their society 'knows' about drunkenness; and accepting and acting upon the understandings thus imparted to them, they become the living confirmation of their society's teachings"* (MacAndrew and Edgerton, 1969, p. 88, emphasis in original).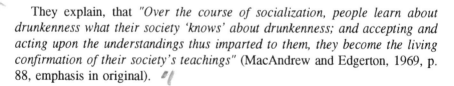

Alcohol Less Important Than Beliefs

Marshall explains that

the pharmacological effects of alcohol on human beings make people *feel* different than when they haven't imbibed. The meanings given to this experience, i.e, how one interprets these feelings and orders his experience, are provided by the culture in which one is a participant. If the culture holds that imbibing alcohol produces warm feelings of community solidarity, harmony, and camaraderie, then violence and sexual advances will have no place (e.g., Brandes 1979). If, on the other hand, the cultural tradition suggests that the drinker will feel aggressive and sexually aroused and, furthermore, will not be held accountable if he acts upon these impulses, then aggression and overt sexual advances are likely to result from drinking (e.g., Hamer 1980). Thus, alcohol as a drug can be viewed as an *enabler* or a *facilitator* of certain culturally given inebriate states, but it cannot be seen as producing a specific response pattern among all human beings who ingest it (Marshall, 1981, p. 200).

Experimental support for this observation is provided by Marlatt and Rohsenow's (1981) work in which they demonstrate that "people will act in certain stereotypical ways when they drink, even if they are drinking tonic water but have been told they are drinking vodka and tonic." For example, men who believed they were drinking vodka (but were only drinking tonic water) became more aggressive. However, when they were drinking vodka but thought it was only tonic water, they did not become more aggressive. Similar effects are found for feelings of anxiety and sexuality.[5]

"Because of our exposure to drinking models presented both in real life and in the media, we have come to expect that people will sometimes do things under the influence of alcohol that they would never do otherwise," Marlatt and Rohsenow (1981) explain. "Alcohol is frequently consumed in relaxed, convivial settings in which sexual advances, for example, are appropriate. In this sense," they write, "alcohol acts as a cue for sexual behavior. The cue effects are the same regardless of the pharmacological properties of alcohol, as long as the people involved believe they are really drinking liquor." Room (1992, p. 103) explains, that "Because intoxication is culturally regarded as causing obstreperous or evil behavior, getting drunk indeed has these effects and, to an extent, legitimates them; a desire to be obstreperous may thus motivate a drunkenness episode."

Alcohol Problems Rare

It is only because of our unique cultural and historical background that we might be surprised to learn, "A major finding, in cross-cultural perspective, is that alcohol-related problems are really rare, even in many societies where drinking is customary, and drunkenness is commonplace" (Heath, 1987, pp. 18-19).

Anthropologists generally agree that "most societies that use alcohol are virtually free of alcohol-related troubles" (Heath, 1987, p. 36) and "few have anything that might be called 'alcoholism' or even frequent 'drinking problems,' even when drinking and drunkenness are common" (Heath, 1987, p. 24). In the words of Mandelbaum (1979, p. 17), "addiction to alcohol seems to be quite rare outside certain societies of Western civilization." More specifically, "The association of drinking with any kind of specifically associated problems--physical, economic, psychological, social relational, or other--is rare among cultures throughout both history and the contemporary world" (Heath, 1987, p. 46).

It has been observed that "solitary, addictive, problem drinking is rare in small traditional societies (Marshall, 1979, p. 451). In fact, "Solitary drinking, often viewed as a crucial symptom of problem drinking, is virtually unknown in most societies" of the world (Heath, 1987, p. 49).

Alcohol Problem Statistics Are Inflated

However, even in the complex industrial United States, the proportion of drinkers who experience serious drinking problems is almost always estimated to be no higher than 10%, even though estimates are often inflated by a diversity of entrepreneurs who have a vested interest in exaggerating the extent of drinking problems. Such entrepreneurs include salvation entrepreneurs, who provide prevention and treatment services; governmental entrepreneurs, whose careers depend upon the perception of widespread serious drinking problems; and moral entrepreneurs, who promote ideological agendas (Mauss, 1991, pp. 190-192; Chauncey, 1980). Anthropologists who report low rates of alcohol problems have even been implicitly accused of "problem deflation" (Room, 1984), a serious threat to entrepreneurs whose careers and income depend upon a widespread public perception of alcohol problems as being numerous, serious, threatening, and growing. Reality tends to recede in salience; it is primarily perception that is important to those with a vested interest. It is not surprising that there appears to be little, if any, correlation between the actual incidence of drinking problems and the levels of funding to fight such problems allocated by governmental bodies in the United States (Mauss, 1991, p. 196).

Harold Mulford (1982, p. 453) has stressed the often enormous discrepancy between official and valid "knowledge."

NIAAA's[6] legislatively mandated reports to Congress contain the official prevalence and distribution data for the nation. They are the most publicized prevalence and distribution conclusions and the ones most often cited by politicians and program policy makers. Their official character, however, is not to be confused with scientific validity. Whether by design or not, the reports to Congress likely reflect a contemporary fact of life. The welfare, perhaps even the survival, of NIAAA, depends upon (1) the apparent magnitude of the alcohol problem, and (2) whether it is made to appear that a disease (rather than a moral or social problem) is being attacked.

He explains that the NIAAA reports use Cahalan's (1970) intentionally very broad definition of problem drinker, which was designed to identify both problem drinkers and *potential* problem drinkers. Not only did his definition include anyone who had experienced a drinking problem within the previous three years, but also anyone who was *likely* to have a problem in the future. "Presenting Cahalan's problem drinker rate as the official rate for the nation, NIAAA, in effect, suddenly nearly doubled the apparent size of the nation's alcoholic population from around 5 million, as had been estimated by the well-known Jellinek formula, to some 9 or 10 million. It is all too easy to conclude from the reports to Congress that there are 10 million Americans suffering a disease requiring medical treatment--a conclusion one might question after studying Cahalan's procedures for identifying problem drinkers" (Mulford, 1982, pp. 453-454), or after learning that Cahalan himself protested the distortion (Wiener, 1981, p. 185) and criticizes this misuse of statistics by lobbyists (Cahalan, 1979,

p. 18).

Other researchers (Gross, 1983, pp. 118-123; Gusfield, 1981, pp. 55-60) have made similar observations regarding the systematic distortion of data by the NIAAA and other governmental agencies. Josephson (1980, p. i) asserts:

An objective assessment of government statistics on alcohol-related problems, many of them compiled in the [NIAAA] *Third Report to the U.S. Congress on Alcohol and Health* in 1978, indicates that there is little sound basis for claims that there are upwards of 10 million problem drinkers (including alcoholics) in the adult population and that their number is increasing; that there are 1.5 to 2.25 million problem drinkers among women; that there are over 3 million problem drinkers among youth; that the heavy consumption of alcohol by pregnant women leads consistently to a cluster of birth defects--the so-called Fetal Alcohol Syndrome; that half of all motor vehicle accident fatalities are alcohol-related; and that the cost of alcohol abuse in 1975 was $43 billion. These and other claims about the extent and consequences of alcohol use and abuse--some of them fanciful, others as yet to be supported by research--are part of the "numbers game" which besets discussion of alcohol-related problems and policy.

For example, the NIAAA estimates of the costs of alcohol abuse are based on highly questionable assumption, confuse statistical association with causality, look only at costs while ignoring benefits (Rice, 1993), are not based on sound accounting procedures and are flawed in numerous other ways, but are presented to Congress and the American public as factual knowledge (Heien and Pittman, 1989, *passim*; Wiener, 1981, pp. 185-188; Ford, 1988, pp. 134-165). The role of alcohol in traffic accidents is similarly exaggerated. For example, Ross and Hughes (1986, p. 663) assert, "It is frequently stated that alcohol is responsible for 50 percent of U.S. traffic fatalities, but the statistic has no solid foundation. The figure includes all traffic deaths in which anyone directly involved has consumed any alcohol. . . . Perhaps the most accurate estimate, from the National Academy of Sciences, attributes roughly 25 percent of fatal accidents to intoxication."

Zylman (1974) has demonstrated how estimates of the number of accidents in which alcohol *might be involved* in any way (passenger, pedestrian, etc.) become transformed into statistics on the number of accidents *caused* by drunk drivers. There appears to be "a need, perhaps even a desire, to blame as many deaths as possible on alcohol" (Zylman, 1974, p. 64).[7] Unfortunately, "estimates take on the status of authoritative facts, disguising their equivocal nature" (Wiener, 1981, p. 184) and thus become enshrined as official truth.

Federal entrepreneurs are not the only ones who have a vested interest in exaggerating the extent of the problem. As Pittman (1988, p. 134) observes, "There are vested economic interests that are trying to expand the definition of alcoholism problems to benefit the treatment industry which has emerged over the last two decades."

While there may be disagreement (and exaggeration) regarding the exact percentage of problem drinkers in the United States or elsewhere, and in the extent of alcohol problems, it is clear around the world that "most of the peoples who drink--like most of the individuals in Western society who drink--do so without suffering in any discernible way" (Heath, 1987, p. 49).[8]

Marshall (1979, p. 452, emphasis his) observes:

Beverage alcohol usually is not a problem in society unless and until it is defined as such. Nonmoralistic attitudes toward alcoholic beverages generally seem to accompany non-pathological uses of such beverages, and vice versa. Yawney [1979], for instance, observes that East Indians in Trinidad, who are ambivalent about alcohol and practice religions opposed to alcohol use, suffer a much higher incidence of alcoholism than blacks in the same country, who accept drinking and drunkenness and adhere to religions that do not moralize about alcohol. One of Lurie's [1979] main points is that the moralistic stances on American Indian drinking adopted by whites have contributed to the perception of a problem where one does not always exist. Westermeyer [1979] . . . reinforces this point, and Lemert [1979] reaches a similar conclusion when commenting on the French view of Society Islanders' drinking and the islanders' own views on the matter. Several writers [in the Marshall anthology] also show that when alcoholic beverages are viewed as a "nonproblem" they usually are not a problem (e.g., Carstairs [1979], Singer [1979], Netting [1979], and Keller [1979]).

Alcohol is used for both secular and religious celebrations the world over, which is an observation frequently made in the literature. Not surprisingly, drinking is usually seen as a pleasant and sociable activity (Marshall, 1979, p. 254).

The anthropological evidence has clearly proven to be helpful in eliminating misconceptions about the use and abuse of alcohol. However, analyses of drinking in groups more widely known to western readers is invaluable in refining our understanding of factors associated with use and misuse of alcohol, especially in our own society. To that end, attention will now be focused on a selection of such groups.

"MODERN" GROUPS

Jews Rarely Abuse Alcohol

Jews constitute a group well-known for the successful ability to enjoy alcohol widely with a minimum of resulting problems. With an amazingly high degree of consistency, research has long demonstrated that, although most Jews drink, they tend to have extremely low rates of alcoholism and other drinking problems. This is true among Jews ranging from Orthodox to Reform, rich to poor, rural to urban, educated to uneducated, and from country to country (Chafetz and Demone, 1962, pp. 84, 86-88; Snyder, 1958, pp. 113-140, 183-202; Snyder and Landman, 1951; Glatt, 1980, p. 192; Skolnick, 1958; Bailey et al., 1965; Ulman, 1960, Unkovic et al., 1980, pp. 179-184; Samuelson, 1878, p. 170; Cahalan,

1970, pp. 53-54, 56, 57, 188; Glassner and Berg, 1985, pp. 94, 102, 104; Schmidt and Popham, 1980, p. 163; Jellinek, 1941a, p. 623; Jellinek, 1941b; Cheinisse, 1908, p. 624; Riley and Marden, 1947; Chafetz, 1964, p. 301). These low rates[9] occur in spite of the fact that Jews would appear to have at least as many fears and anxieties, often viewed as causing drinking problems, as do others (Glatt, 1980, pp. 188-190; Wilkinson, 1970, pp. 20 and 23). Snyder (1962, p. 188) observed that "there is no lack among Jews of acute psychic tensions of the sort which are popularly supposed to cause drinking pathologies" and stressed, "In comparison to certain other groups exhibiting an excess of alcohol problems, perhaps it may be said that they have an undue share of anxieties which have their origin in broad social and historical circumstances." Empirical research (for example, Bales, 1946, p. 490; Fein, 1958, p. 101; and Hyde and Chisholm, 1944, p. 617; Knupfer and Room, 1967) supports this position. The heterogeneity of Jews in terms of genetic background, or physical or "racial" characteristics reduces the credibility of any biologically based explanation (Snyder, 1962, pp. 188-189). A second problem with a genetic explanation is that drunkenness appears to have been frequent among Jews during the age of the Prophets but then virtually disappeared after the return from the first Babylonian exile (about 600 B.C.) (Keller, 1970, pp. 290-292; Weber, 1952, pp. 188-189). Because no genetic change could have occurred, the answer would appear to lie elsewhere.

Bales has identified the Orthodox Jewish attitude toward drinking as ritualistic. The bases for this orientation begin early. When he is only eight days old the Orthodox boy is circumcised, signifying his entry into the covenant between Jehovah and the Jewish people. Additionally, first-born sons experience the redemption rite thirty days after birth. This ceremony also ordinarily involves the ritual use of wine (Snyder, 1958, p. 21).

The first religious education involves teaching the proper benedictions for food and drink (Bales, 1946, p. 491). "The child is to be instructed by law in the rituals of drinking at the earliest possible age" (Skolnick, 1957, p. 66). "In the Jewish culture wine stands for a whole complex of sacred things. Wine is variously alluded to as 'the word of God' and 'the commandment of the Lord.' Similarly, the Torah (the sacred body of the Law), Jerusalem (the sacred lace), Israel (the sacred community), and 'the Messiah' (the righteous) are all compared to wine" (Bales, 1946, p. 491).

The ritual attitude toward drinking "requires that alcoholic beverages, sometimes a particular one, should be used in the performance of religious ceremonies. Typically the beverage is regarded as sacred, it is consecrated to that end, and the partaking of it is a ritual act of communion with the sacred" (Bales, 1946, p. 487). Wine is not only used ritually on the sabbath but it is also significant in the annual cycle of holy days and festivals.

While there is no special use of wine or alcoholic beverages at the Bar Mitzvah, these beverages are sanctified and used as a part of the celebration meal (Snyder, 1958, p. 32). Another very important rite of passage is marriage, and drinking plays a role in the wedding ceremony. During this ceremony the rabbi utters the benediction over a cup of wine and hands it to the bridal couple, who drink it. They may then pass it to their nearest relatives, who also drink. It is also customary for the groom to break a wine glass on the floor or to crush it with his feet (Snyder, 1958, pp. 32-33).

Between death and the time of burial, mourning requires abstention from meat and wine (except during holy days). Furthermore, the *Schulchan Aruch* requires that the head of the deceased be washed with wine (Snyder, 1958, p. 33).

It is Bales' belief that

[i]n the Jewish culture the wine is sacred and drinking is an act of communion. The act is repeated again and again and the attitudes toward drinking are all bound up with attitudes toward the sacred in the mind and emotions of the individual. In my opinion this is the central reason why drunkenness is regarded as so "indecent"--so unthinkable--for a Jew. Rational precaution also probably plays a part, but the ritual use is the main mechanism which builds in the necessary emotional support for the attitudes. Drunkenness is a profanity, an abomination, a perversion of the sacred use of wine. Hence the idea of drinking "to become drunk" for some individualistic or selfish reason arouses a counteranxiety so strong that very few Jews ever become compulsive drinkers (1946, p. 493).

Similarly, Thorner (1953, p. 175) has written that in Orthodox Judaism "the physiological and psychological effects of alcohol are incidental to rituals symbolizing, communicating and strengthening religious and social sentiments." In fact, "Sobriety is a standard, among others, by which the degree of fulfillment of obligations to God and the Jewish community may be determined" (Snyder, 1962, p. 217).

Jews Learn How Not to Drink

Jews learn how to drink properly by example and experience in the home and they simultaneously learn how *not* to drink. For example, the common ditty "Shikker iz a Goy" (Drunkard is a Gentile), implies that drunkenness is un-Jewish (Snyder, 1958, pp. 158-161):

The Gentile goes into the saloon, the saloon,
And drinks there a small glass of wine;
  he tosses it off--his glass of wine.
Oh--the Gentile is a Drunkard--a drunkard he is,
Drink he must,
Because he is a Gentile!
The Gentile comes into our alley, our little street,
And breaks the windows of us poor Jews;
  our windowpanes are broken out,
For--the Gentile is a Drunkard--a drunkard he is,

Drink he must,
Because he is a Gentile!
The Jew hurries into the place of prayer;
An evening prayer, a short benediction he says,
  and a prayer for his dead.
For--the Jew is a sober man--sober is he,
Pray he must,
Because he is a Jew. (Translated by Bales, 1944, pp. 136-137.)

Sobriety is considered a Jewish virtue, while drunkenness is a Gentile vice (Zimberg, 1977, p. 574; Blaine, 1980, p. 9; Unkovic et al., 1980, pp. 169 and 184; Zimberg, 1980, p. 208; Glassner and Berg, 1985, p. 95). Consequently, while Gentiles are expected to become drunk, Jews who do so are subject to scorn[10] as expressed in the well-known Jewish folk saying, "A Yid a Shikker, zoll geharget veren!" ("A Jew who's a drunkard, may he get killed") (Snyder, 1962, p. 217).

Blacker has summarized that Jews begin to drink at a very early age. They also tend to drink frequently and to consume a variety of alcoholic beverages. The settings for consumption are diverse. But in all cases moderation is encouraged. Drunkenness is rare, inappropriate intoxicated behavior is sanctioned and most Jews agree with the disapproval. There is an absence of emotionalism or ambivalence associated with the moderate use of alcohol (1966, pp. 60-61).

The farther the Jew is from the Orthodox tradition, the greater the likelihood of intemperate drinking (Meystel, 1949, p. 149). As religious affiliation shifts from Orthodox to Conservative to Reform and to Secular, there is a systematic (although still very low) increase in the incidence of drinking problems (Snyder, 1962, p. 190; Snyder, 1958, p. 125; Snyder et al., 1982, pp. 638 and 651). In Snyder's (1962, p. 190) words, "intoxication and signs of more extreme drinking pathologies are conspicuous by their absence among more Orthodox, despite their extensive use of wines, spirits, and beers. However, as religion shifts from Orthodox to Conservative to Reform to Secular, signs of drinking pathologies show marked and systematic increases." However, Glassner and Berg (1985, pp. 96-97) found such increases to be very low. They believe that the moral symbolism reinforced through group rites need not be only religious; their interviews suggest to them that it can be achieved "by restricting drinking to special secular occasions and by cataloguing drinking as a symbolic part of festive eating" (Glassner and Berg, 1985, p. 97). Less religious Jews are also more likely to be problem drinkers (Unkovic et al., 1980, pp. 181-184; Jones, 1963, pp. 23-24; Patai, 1980, pp. 80-81; Glatt, 1980, pp. 194 and 200), although in their study of 29 Jewish alcoholics, Schmidt and Popham (1980, p. 163) failed to find support for that generalization.

Unkovic and his colleagues (1980, p. 184) identified the following as the most significant factors contributing to Jewish sobriety:

1) The solidarity of the Jewish community.
2) Emotionally sustained tradition and family organization.
3) The fact that wine is a religious symbol and is first drunk early in life.
4) The fact that alcoholism would be disruptive to the unity of the Jewish people.
5) The religious teachings of Judaism regulate alcoholic consumption.
6) Sobriety is a Jewish virtue.

Snyder (1958, p. 202) concluded, "Where drinking is an integral part of the socialization process, where it is interrelated with the central moral symbolism and is repeatedly practiced in the rites of the group, the phenomenon of alcoholism is conspicuous by its absence. Norms of sobriety can be effectively sustained under these circumstances even though the drinking is extensive." He stressed that, on the other hand, "Where institutional conflicts disrupt traditional patterns in which drinking is integrated, where drinking is dissociated from the normal process of socialization, where drinking is relegated to social contexts which are disconnected from or in opposition to the core moral values and where it is used for individual purposes, pathologies such as alcoholism may be expected to increase" (Snyder, 1958, p. 202).

Irish Suffer High Alcohol Abuse

Early Christians adopted many of the same drinking norms as did the Jews, although there was less emphasis upon wine as a sacred symbol. While Jesus drank wine in both ritual and non-ritual contexts, both he and the Apostle Paul warned against drunkenness. At the present time the only Christian religious ritual in which wine is used is that of the celebration of the Last Supper (Fitzpatrick, 1963, pp. 13-14). Furthermore, not all Christian groups use wine in that ritual.

The official Roman Catholic view is that total abstinence (except for religious communion) is desirable and virtuous, especially if practiced for a motive such as penance, good example, reparation for sins or safeguarding sobriety. On the other hand, drinking in moderation is approved. It is argued, "Alcohol is neither morally good nor morally bad; it is morally indifferent, or morally neutral in itself" (Ford, 1961, p. 51). However, drunkenness is considered immoral, as it impairs a person's reason and judgment and prevents the mind from being turned toward God (Fitzpatrick, 1963, pp. 14-15).

While the above appears to be the formal Roman Catholic position, it is important to note that the Church is not so monolithic as it may at first appear and that considerable variation in practice occurs, especially from nation to nation. For example, Bales (1962, pp. 163-164) has pointed out that the Irish secular norms are in direct conflict with the official position of the Church. Historically, the rural Irish clergy were recruited from the people and supported by the people, and it is not strange that their attitudes toward drinking were similar to those of their parishioners. "The practical attitude of the Irish clergy generally was tolerant and permissive, occasionally interrupted with protests, but just as often veering into a more or less complete participation in the drinking customs of the people" (Bales, 1962, p. 164).

Stivers (1976, p. 1) asserts that "students of drink have all come to the conclusion that among white American ethnic groups, no group has given evidence of a greater tendency toward drunkenness and alcoholism than the Irish."[11]

Current Irish attitudes and practices regarding alcohol can be traced back to the last century in rural Ireland. The first passage rite for the Irish infant was, and is, baptism, a Roman Catholic sacrament which is believed to make possible entry into heaven. In part to maintain family status, the parents would be expected to provide liberal amounts of whisky and/or other alcoholic beverages to those who attend the baptism; this drinking was not part of the ritual and has no religious significance (Bales, 1944, p. 154).

Irish children go to their first confession soon after beginning to attend school. After going to confession for some time they are given special instruction preparing them for their first communion. In this important rite, the wine is believed to become the blood of Christ. The symbolism of communion is virtually equivalent to the Jewish Kiddush at Passover in that it signifies a union with the sacred. Traditionally, however, there is one very important difference: only the priest partakes of the wine (Bales, 1944, pp. 170-171).

Bales argues that, for several reasons, the consumption of wine in holy communion is not associated in the mind of the Irish with drinking in the usual sense of that word. One reason is that the laity does not partake of wine[12] in the Irish culture as it does in the Jewish. A second is that the Jewish child is taught the relevant sacred ideas and attitudes at an earlier age and within the familiar environment of the family. A third is that the Irish child is exposed to non-ritual uses of drinking earlier and in much greater frequency than is the Jewish child. A fourth reason is that sacramental wine is seen as being very different because it is the only permissible substance for the ritual, whereas in Jewish culture any beverage other than water is acceptable for the Kiddush. Thus, "the attitudes applying to the wine used in the ritual are also expected to apply to other alcoholic beverages in the Jewish culture, whereas in the Irish culture they are not" (Bales, 1944, pp. 171-172; also see Patai, 1980, pp. 72-73).

Young people in Ireland are confirmed somewhere between the ages of 12 and 15. Religiously, this passage rite marks their transition to active membership in the Church; socially it marks their transition into a semi-adult world of increasing work and responsibility. No alcohol is used in this important rite (Bales, 1944, p. 179).

The fact that confirmation marks "semi-adulthood" in Ireland is important. This failure to achieve adulthood at confirmation existed not only in the last century but was also documented as the mid-twentieth century approached

(Arensberg and Kimball, 1940). Father and sons work together tilling small farms, and a son cannot marry until his father has turned the farm over to him. Bales (1944, p. 179-180) explained, "Until that time the son is called a 'boy,' and has the social status of a boy, no matter how old he may be." Thus, "Fathers of 'boys' of 45 and 50 collect any wages they may earn at day labor elsewhere, and the 'boy' must look to his father for direction, advice, and even spending money" (Bales, 1944, p. 180).

Not only are males required to be submissive to their fathers, but they are also required to be segregated from females (Kennedy, 1973, p. 172). And this separation in both work and leisure continues after marriage. Drinking and male companionship are encouraged and function to preserve the status quo. Thus, male identity came to be associated with hard drinking (Stivers, 1985, p. 111; 1976, p. 67). He who does not spend his free time drinking with the boys is suspect; perhaps he is getting a girl pregnant or otherwise ruining her reputation. An anthropologist reported hearing that the teetotaler is a menace to society, and another writer reported hearing "from responsible Irish people that the danger to society lies not in the drunkard . . . but with the teetotaler" (de la Fontaine, 1940, p. 32 quoted in Bales, 1944, p. 182). Men are encouraged to sublimate their sexuality through drinking and to deal with any emotional problems by "drinking it off." On the basis of his case records, Bales contended that the encouragement of drinking to solve problems has been preserved in Irish-American culture (Bales, 1944, p. 183; 1962, p. 169).

Not surprisingly,

the drunkard in Ireland is not condemned, unless he is married and his drinking threatens the family's cash resources or tenure on the land, when he is said to "go to town and drink the money," or "drink the land up," leaving nothing for his parents, siblings, or children (39). Where drunkenness begins to interfere with the primary family system and its economic base, rather than facilitate its preservation, it is condemned. Short of that, drunkenness, as Arensberg says, is "laughable, pleasurable, somewhat exciting, a punctuation of dull routine to be watched and applauded, and drunken men are handled with care and affection" (39). The drunkard is handled with maternal affection, often referred to as the poor "boy," with a special connotation of sympathy, love, pity, and sorrow. If married, the drunkard is compassionately classed by his wife with "the min, God help us!" (45, p. 87). The man who is drunk is sometimes regarded with envy by the man who is sober. (Bales, 1962, p. 170).

Attitudes toward immoderate drinking continues to be tolerant in contemporary Ireland (Armyr et al., 1982, p. 63). "The typical attitude towards [problem] drinking is illustrated by the alleged opposition on the part of trade unions to attempts to detect alcoholics among industrial workers for the purpose of early treatment. Doctors are often said to provide humorously worded sick-notes to patients unable to report for work because of a hangover. Absenteeism from work, particularly on Mondays, because of drinking problems is regarded as a normal occurrence." Not surprisingly, alcohol-related psychiatric and other problems continue to occur frequently among Irish men (Brody, 1973; Scheper-Hughes, 1970; McGoldrick, 1982). A study in New York State psychiatric facilities of alcohol-related diagnoses revealed that 51.3% of Irish male immigrants were hospitalized for such diagnoses, compared to only 13.8% for all male immigrants; 11.8% of Irish female immigrants were admitted with alcohol-related diagnoses, compared to only 2.6% for all female immigrants (Muhlin, 1985, p. 173).

On the basis of his research, Glad (1947) concluded, "Jews tend to regard the function of drinking as (a) socially practical and (b) religiously symbolic and communicative. The common element in these two uses lies in their instru-mentality to the attainment of goals remote from the effects of alcohol per se. The Irish tend to regard the functions of drinking as (a) promotion of fun and pleasure and (b) conviviality. Both of these define the purpose of drinking in terms of effective consequences, in which the physiological and psychological changes produced in the individual by alcohol per se are of primary importance."

Most Italians Drink, Few Abuse

Italians have also long been identified as a group whose members generally drink and who consume at a high level, but who are characterized with a low level of alcoholism or other drinking problems (Lolli et al., 1958, p. xii; Rorabaugh, 1979, p. 239; New York State Bureau of Drug Addiction, 1980, p. 36-37; Straus and Bacon, 1953; Unkovic et al., 1980, p. 171; Ulman, 1960; Garvin, 1930; Moros, 1942; Greeley and McCready, 1975; Greeley et al., 1980, pp. 38-45; Haggard and Jellinek, 1942; Jellinek, 1951). In the words of Greeley et al. (1980, pp. 38-39), "The Irish are heavy drinkers with serious [drinking] problems, Italians are heavy drinkers with a minimum of serious problems."

The vast majority of Italians are first exposed to alcohol as part of their regular family, social or religious life; they drink (often exclusively) with regular meals; their shared experience of drinking reflects a cohesion or a sociability rather than a means to achieve it; very few drink for the physiological effect; most take alcohol for granted and have no strong feelings about it; and they consider moderate amounts of wine to be acceptable for children to drink (Lolli et al., 1958, pp. 65, 70, 71, 73 and 82).

Describing life in an Italian village, Moss and Cappannari (1960, p. 96) wrote, "Large amounts of poor quality wine are used to wash down food; though the wine is low in alcohol content (10%-11%), copious amounts are taken. Drunkenness is rare and alcoholism is virtually unknown."

Simboli (1985, p. 65) observed that Italians view wine as healthful. "Further evidence of cultural integration of wine is the fact that children drink wine with their parents in public places."[13] He continued (p. 65):

Home winemaking by many Italian-Americans also indicates wine's importance as a cultural focus. The art of home winemaking involves deep-rooted beliefs that link land and family social organization through viticulture. It takes years of patient care to raise vines so that they can produce a quality grape for the production of wine. It also takes the combined effort of family members and friends to harvest the grapes and make the wine. Great care is taken to ensure that wine does not spoil while it is aging. Proper aging ensures a "healthy" wine, which also means that the body consuming it will be healthy.

Summarizing the research by Lolli and his colleagues of drinking among Italians, Keller (1958, p. xiv) asserted that "for Italians drinking is a part of eating, even a form of eating, for wine is a food; that to the extent that the descendants of Italians in America retain ancestral cultural traditions, they drink with the same attitudes and in the same ways; and that the set of attitudes which does not separate drink from food is at least partly responsible for the relative sobriety of Italian drinking." In the words of another writer, "Drinking in Italy, is a social event centered around the meal. Wine is a food to be used with meals" (Morgan, 1982, p. 15; also see Jellinek, 1962, p. 388). While there is low pressure to drink (for example, one can refuse a drink without offending), drunkenness carries negative social sanctions (Blacker, 1966, p. 60).

When it occurs, intoxication tends to occur in mixed-gender groups where it is subject to appropriate social controls. (This is in contrast to Irish men, who tend to become intoxicated in bars in the company of other men only) (Chafetz and Demone, 1962, p. 83).

Lolli and his colleagues found rates of intoxication among Italians to be low. Importantly, "the proportion of subjects who had never experienced intoxication was substantially higher among Italians than among Italian-Americans" (Lolli et al., 1958, p. 83). More precisely, the proportion who had ever experienced intoxication was 38% among Italians, 49% among first-generation Italian-Americans, and 66% among than of the second or third generation (Lolli et al., 1958, p. 83). The same phenomenon was reported by Jessor et al. (1970, p. 218), who found from 42% to 48% of their respondents in Italy having been "drunk or pretty high" at least once in the last year, while 76% of their Italian-American respondents had been in that condition in the last year. On the basis of his research, Simboli (1985, pp. 72-73) concluded that "drinking behavior among Italian-Americans is directly related to generational membership group and is not just an artifact of age or social position and with more acculturation[14] into American society, drinking practices change significantly and with a concomitant increase in problem drinking."

As Italian-Americans drop the traditional attitudes and behaviors concerning alcohol, they begin to lose the protection of the Italian drinking tradition and begin to exhibit more drinking problems. But their rate of problems remains significantly below that of other Americans in general (Blane, 1977; Chafetz and Demone, 1962, p. 83-84). While in his small sample, Salvatore (1979, p. 14) found that the percentage of peak drinkers (those consuming five or more drinks on any given occasion) declined with succeeding generations, Greeley and his colleagues have demonstrated that the drinking subcultures of Italian-Americans (as well as that of Irish-Americans) are "remarkably durable" across generations (Greeley et al., 1980, p. 91).

Clear differences in alcoholism rates between foreign-born and American-born soldiers of Italian and Irish background are apparent in Table 2.1. Among the Italians, the alcoholism rate is lower among the foreign-born, while among the Irish it is those born in this country who have a lower rate.

Vaillant (1986, p. 147) reported substantial differences between second-generation men over the age of 40, as seen in Table 2.2. He also found (using the DSM-III [American Psychiatric Association, 1980] diagnostic criteria) that "[a]lcohol dependence developed seven times more frequently in the Irish than those [of] Mediterranean descent," the difference being 28% to 4% (Vaillant, 1986, p. 147).

TABLE 2.1
Total Neuropsychiatric Cases in Foreign and American-Born Soldiers of Italian and Irish Stock and Percentage "Alcoholic" of Italian and Irish in Each Group in World War I

Ethnic Group	Total Neuro-Psychiatric Cases	Percentage "Alcoholic"
Italian		
Foreign-Born	2,039	0.2
American-Born	413	1.2
Irish		
Foreign-Born	394	18.0
American-Born	4,068	9.4

Note - Adapted from Glad (1947, p. 26).

Blacker summarized the common characteristics of the Jews and the Italians, both groups with low rates of alcoholism as

1) gradual socialization of children in the use of alcoholic beverages;
2) relatively low social pressure to drink;
3) negative sanctions against excessive drinking;
4) positive, accepting attitudes toward moderate, non-disruptive drinking;
5) a well-established consensus on the customs of drinking; and
6) freedom from ambivalence in the drinking situation (1966, p. 62).

TABLE 2.2
Ethnicity and Reported Drinking Problems (in Percent)

Problem	Irish ($\underline{n}$ = 76)	Mediterranean[a] ($\underline{n}$ = 128)
Wife complains	22	10
Multiple medical problems	12	0
Clinical diagnosis of alcoholism	17	2
Multiple drunkenness arrests	26	5
Multiple hospitalizations for alcoholism	16	2
8+ problems	26	3

Note - Adapted from Vaillant (1986, p. 147).

[a] Includes men from Italy, Portugal, Spain, Greece, Syria, and Armenia and six Jews in the sample (Vaillant, 1986, p. 143).

Chinese Drink with Few Problems

The Chinese have long been recognized as a group that uses alcohol in moderation and that experiences very few drinking problems. Based on his experience as a social worker in Peking between 1934 and 1937, Hsu (1970, p. 67) observed that alcoholism is as "rare in China as it appears to be abundant in the United States." LaBarre's experience in China during World War II led him to write, "The Chinese are not so voluntarily addicted to excessive use of alcohol as have been some northern European peoples. . . ." He continued, "The fact seems to be that in spite of ample and even copious consumption of alcohol on defined occasions, its use appears never to become an emotional problem." (LaBarre, 1946, p. 375). In a seventeen-year period, no more than ten cases of alcoholism were reported among the Chinese population of Taiwan (Chafetz, 1964, p. 298).

More recent writers have made similar observations. For example, the London *Times'* Peking Bureau chief (Bonavia, 1980, p. 279) described the "near absence of alcoholism" and public drunkenness in China in spite of the fact that "the shelves of the liquor counters in department stores positively groan under the weight of multicolored brews" and the vast majority of ordinary Chinese people drink at least occasionally. Reporting on his three-week tour of China, an alcohol researcher (Schaefer, 1980, p. 19) described "the absence of alcohol abuse" and speculated, "The family and neighborhood/commune peer pressure on most decisions is probably a key to the feeling that excess will not be tolerated." Systematic studies corroborate such observations. For example, an epidemiologic survey in a Taiwanese town of 19,931 inhabitants identified only two alcoholics (Lin, 1953) and, among Chinese Americans, the death rates from chronic liver disease and alcoholic cirrhosis is only about one-fourth that of white Americans (Yu and Liu, 1986/87, p. 16). While Indians and Chinese in Singapore aged 15 and above drink the same quantities with the same frequency, the alcoholism rate for Chinese is only about 5% that of the Indians (*Medical Gazette*, 1987, p. 88 cited in Isralowitz and Hong, 1988, 1321).

Chinese-born residents of New York City's Chinatown reported (Barnett, 1955, p. 186-187) that in China, drinking[15] was very much a part of the daily routine. Children were introduced to wine during meals at an early age. "The children drank and watched others drink at social gatherings, at religious ceremonies, in the market place, and in their own households" (Barnett, 1955, p. 186). Through their experience and observation, children learned a set of attitudes about the practice. "While drinking was socially sanctioned, becoming drunk was not" (Barnett, 1955, p. 186). Confucian and Taoist philosophies in China emphasized the need for moderation in drinking alcohol (Helzer et al., 1990, p. 317; Heok, 1990, p. 571; Culver, 1987, p. 20; Royce, 1986, p. 57; Singer, 1974). Individuals who lost control of themselves because of intoxication were ridiculed and, if they persisted in their defection, were ostracized. Their lack of moderation was considered to be not only a personal shortcoming, but also a deficiency of the entire family. While second-generation parents in Chinatown had become more acculturated to American beliefs, drinking still played an important role in their lives and there was no condemnation of drinking in moderation (Barnett, 1955, pp. 186-187).

An example of social sanction among Chinese-Americans was provided by Barnett (1955, p. 202):

At a late supper there was heavy drinking. A younger man . . . became quite intoxicated and fell asleep. One of the party dashed out of the hall and returned with a camera and flash equipment. He took a photograph of the recumbent figure. The following day, on the bulletin board used by this group there was posted a print of the offender. The upper part of his body was slouched over the table. The face had been cut out so that identification was difficult. Underneath was a hand-printed caption stating that here was the picture of a man who drank too much and didn't know how to control himself. If he persisted in disgracing his friends the same print would appear--with the face included.

Condemnation of drunkenness has been systematically documented in surveys of Chinese-Americans (Chu, 1972).

According to Chinese folk belief, excessive use of alcohol brings on "ninefold harm": (1) it impairs the intellect, (2) it impairs morals, (3) it leads to physical illness, (4) it impairs sexual performance, (5) it shortens the lifespan, (6) it impairs fertility, (7) it leads to the transmission of inherited defects, (8) it increases the risk of suicide, and (9) it increases criminality (Yu et al., 1985, p. 331). Consuming a drink is viewed as warming the body, but getting intoxicated is seen as burning out the system (Barnett, 1955, p. 198).

It might be noted that Chinese drinking games involve requiring the "loser" to drink; one attempts to remain sober while getting others drunk (Barnett, 1955, pp. 188-189).

Recent studies of Chinese in China, Taiwan, Singapore and the United States (Pai, 1991, pp, 40-42; Helzer et al., 1990; Chi et al., 1988, pp. 24-25; Chi et al., 1989, p. 15; Akutsu et al., 1989, p. 264; Ahern, 1985,[16] p. 324; Yu et al., 1985, p. 339; Yu and Liu, 1986/1987, pp. 16-17; Isralowitz and Hong, 1988, p. 1321; Kitano and Chi, 1985, p. 381; LeMarchand et al., 1985, p. 355) indicate that most drink in moderation, many choose not to drink and very few experience any drinking problems. In their study of Chinese in Los Angeles, Kitano and Chi (1985, p. 381) noted that much drinking by Chinese was done with friends and on special occasions (much as weddings and anniversaries) where there were social controls on their drinking behavior. However, when traditional alcohol beliefs and practices decrease among the Chinese, it appears that they tend to experience a higher incidence of drinking problems and abuse (Yeh and Kwu, 1984, cited in Yu and Liu, 1986/1987, p. 61; Yu and Liu, 1986/1987, p. 61; Sue et al., 1979) almost without exception (Sue et al., 1985, p. 362).

It should be mentioned that since 1972, when Wolff (1972) reported differences in alcohol sensitivity, researchers have studied the "oriental flushing reflex." Large proportions of various oriental populations experience a reddening of the skin, more rapid breathing and an increase in heart rate after drinking alcohol,[17] while only as small percentage of Caucasians do (Kitano, 1989, p. 146). However, no significant relationship has been found between flushing and reported drinking patterns (Sue et al., 1985, cited by Kitano, 1989, p. 146). Because the flushing phenomenon appears to be physiological in origin, it cannot credibly explain differences in alcohol patterns over time or between generations.

The New York State Bureau of Drug Addiction (1980, pp. 17-46) concluded that for groups most of whose members use alcohol, the lowest incidence of alcoholism is found in those groups in which:

1) Children are exposed to diluted alcohol early in life within a strong family or religious setting.
2) The beverage is considered mainly as a food and usually consumed with meals.
3) Parents present an example of moderate drinking.
4) Drinking is considered neither a virtue nor a sin.
5) Drinking is not a sign of adulthood.
6) Abstinence is socially acceptable.
7) Intoxication is not socially acceptable.
8) "Ground rules" of drinking are clear.

Available evidence (for example Straus and Bacon, 1953, p. 49; Skolnick, 1957, pp. 182, 201, 291; Maddox, 1962, p. 239; Pullman, 1958, pp. 627-631; Lawrence and Maxwell, 1962, p. 142) suggests that differences in socioeconomic status are inadequate to explain differences in alcohol use and abuse between religious and cultural groups. However, there is much evidence (Snyder, 1962, pp. 194-195 and 202; Lolli et al., 1958, pp. 83-85; Skolnick, 1957, p. 285; Williams and Straus, 1950, p. 54) that drinking patterns change or individuals interact with those of religious or cultural backgrounds stressing difficult drinking norms. This suggests that it is normative differences associated with specific religious or cultural groups which at least largely influences drinking patterns.

Wilkinson identified five elements common to those cultural drinking patterns that lead to low rates of drinking problems (1970, pp. 6-8). The first is a low level of emotionalism and a lack of ambivalence about drinking. Alcohol is not a major issue. It is not seen as either the key to personal, social or economic success on the one hand or as the share "demon rum" on the other.

Second, there is a clear distinction between drinking per se and drunkenness or other alcohol abuse. A stigma on moderate drinking tends to be counterproductive by inadvertently encouraging exaggerated drinking behavior. It also makes it difficult to provide clear guidelines for young people on how to deal with alcohol in a moderate way. On the other hand, there are taboos on the abuse of alcohol.

Third, drinking occurs in "situations of restraint, that is, when the social atmosphere is such that drunkenness is felt to be out of the question" (Wilkinson, 1970, p. 7).

Fourth, drinking occurs in situations in which it is only one of several integrated activities and does not become an overwhelming focus of the group's attention. Drinking is not a "big deal," abstainers are comfortable not drinking and no one is pressured to drink more than they really want to.

Fifth, drinking often occurs with meals.

Mormon Drinkers Are at Very High Risk

In contrast to most religious organizations, the Church of Jesus Christ of Latterday Saints ("Mormon" Church) prohibits drinking alcohol by its members (Brown, 1963, p. 25). Not surprisingly, a negative relationship between drinking and religious participation was found among Mormons in Straus and Bacon's (1953, p. 51) nation-wide study of college students. Clearly, Mormons who did not drink could not experience drinking problems. However, among those Mormons who did drink, there was a very high incidence of drinking problems, as can been seen in Table 2.3.

A study of over 8,500 students (85% of whom were Mormon) at 19 high schools in Utah similarly found that about half of the junior and senior class users of alcohol had experienced at least one incident of intoxication, and 41.4% of all drinkers had been high or tight during the previous month. Fighting when drinking was more common among students whose parents were abstainers (31.2%) than among those whose parents drank (Jones, 1957, pp. 16, 20 and 40).

At the time Skolnick conducted his 1957 study, the Methodist Church maintained a total abstinence position. Historically, it had been the most strongly organized and influential of the "temperance" (i.e., abstinence) religious groups (Skolnick, 1958, p. 453). Skolnick found a negative relationship between

TABLE 2.3
Incidence of Intoxication by Religion for Male Students Who Drink (in Percent)

		Those who have ever		
By religion	Been tight	Been drunk	Passed out	Been drunk more than five times
Jewish	67	45	18	9
Catholic	73	56	33	15
Protestant	84	68	34	17
Mormon	88	74	40	25

Note - Adapted from Straus and Bacon (1953, p. 136).

drinking and religious participation among his Methodist respondents. More specifically, he (1957, pp. 305-308) found that 65% of the Methodist abstainers participated in religious activities at least once a week, while only 34% of those who drank participated to this degree. Seventy-eight percent of the Methodist and Nazarene[18] abstainers attended church regularly, while only 39% of the drinkers attended regularly. Of the users, only 36% considered themselves to be either fairly or very active in church affairs, while 72% of the abstainers considered themselves to be that active. Importantly, Methodists who violated their church's prohibition against drinking were much more likely to become intoxicated than were Jews, as indicated in Table 2.4.

TABLE 2.4
The Relationship Between Religious Affiliation and Intoxication (Among Those Who Drink)

By Religion	Those who have been intoxicated in any way	Those who have been intoxicated more than five times
Methodist	83	61
Jewish	45	15

Note - Adapted from Skolnick (1957, pp. 198-200).

In his study of over 500 adolescents (Preston, 1969) discovered that those affiliated with churches proscribing alcohol and considering its use a moral problem were more likely to experience drinking problems if they chose to drink. In a study of 3,696 students from 36 colleges across the United States, Hanson (1972; 1978, p. 34) found that drinkers from abstinence backgrounds were more likely to be aggressive and to experience drinking problems. Smith's (1969, p. 26) study of about 5,000 sociology students (about half of whom were Mormons) from two universities similarly found that drinkers affiliated with religious groups teaching abstinence were much more likely to become drunk. A study of 700 tenth grade students found that drinkers who self-identified with religious groups proscribing alcohol were more likely to be heavy drinkers (Hogan, 1979, p. 74). "With respect to social effects, the proscriptive subjects who drank experienced more problems with authority as well as more interpersonal and psychological problems" (p. vi). A study of over 1,800 Native Americans in 20 communities located in ten states (Moss and Janzen, 1980) found that Mormon drinkers were significantly more likely to drink to the point of intoxication than were others.

Armor et al. (1978) found that drinkers from more abstentious groups (Protestants, residents of southern and midwestern states, blacks, and those of lower socioeconomic states) were more likely to become alcoholic. A geographic analysis by Albrecht (1985) drew similar conclusions regarding the alcoholism rate. Davies and Stacey's (1972) research in Scotland suggests that young people who drank heavily tended to have learned more negative beliefs about alcohol and the dangers of alcohol. In her study of data from three national surveys of drinking, Seifert (1972, p. 126) found that, among members of highly abstinent Protestant groups who chose to drink, high proportions engaged in binge drinking and experienced drinking problems.

In his "Prohibition Norms and Teenage Drinking," Globetti (1978, p. 161) reports the nature of drinking among high school students in "a relatively small Mississippi community which represents the prototype of the abstinence cultural attitude." The community is homogeneous in terms of those religious groups which strongly censure drinking. "Imbibing among the students in this locality is not only an illegal activity, as defined by state law, but also a taboo one." A substantial number of students who had discussed drinking and alcohol use with their parents or other adults said that the information given emphasized the evil nature of alcohol.

Globetti (p. 162) found that while only 40% of the students used alcohol, "These drinkers usually were introduced to alcohol outside the home and continued to secure their beverages from a bootlegger or other illegal sources. They drank without parental knowledge and approval, most frequently in a sub-rosa situation with their age peers, and they were not governed by agencies which ordinarily affect restraint. Over 60% reported that they had experienced drinking problems, such as getting in fights, destroying property, experiencing blackouts, or damaging friendships." This compared to a five to ten percent of adolescents who typically report such problems. Globetti concluded that while less drinking can be expected in an abstinence setting, more drinking problems can be expected among those who choose to drink.

Cahalan and Room (1974, p. 172) discovered that "it is in the dry areas [of the U.S.] with a strong abstinence tradition that explosive drinking patterns, social disruptions associated with drinking and acute alcohol poisonings [Room, 1971] predominate." Smith and Hanham (1982, p. 52) observed, "These data support an 'inoculation' theory of drinking, which suggests that excessive or 'binge' drinking might be reduced if the local norms pertaining to drinking were more liberal. In other words, if people were able to drink in a more 'normal' and leisurely fashion, the tendency to drink in bursts might be lessened. The abstaining milieu might also provide a 'breeding' ground for 'very heavy' drinking by forcing drinkers to bunch their drinking to offset the overall lack of availability."

India promotes abstention and, while the percentage of drinkers is low, it appears (Singh, 1979, pp. 522-523) that the percentage of those who drink heavily is high.

Mäkelä (1978) found that in areas of the United States where alcohol consumption is low relative to national norms, indicator rates for problem drinking (especially public drunkenness) tend to be higher than expected. Room (1983, p. 587) found that in those regions of the U.S. with "dryer cultural environments" there were more problems due to drinking at any given level of consumption.

Linsky and his colleagues (Linsky et al., 1986) computed a proscriptive norm index for each of the 50 states based on percentage of the population living in legally dry areas, the degree of legal restrictions on the sale or consumption of alcoholic beverages and the percentage of Mormons and Fundamentalists in the population. They found that there was less drinking in proscriptive states, but that the drinking that did occur tended to be more disruptive. This was so even after controlling for educational level, poverty, metropolitan population, non-white population and age. They conclude (p. 391) that "proscriptive normative systems are significantly correlated with all of the indicators of disruptive alcohol-related behavior. States that have the strongest cultural biases against beverage alcohol tend to be the same states that experience the most problems (i.e., the highest arrest rates associated with drinking)." It is their observation (p. 392) that "societies that fear alcohol soon encounter problems with disruptive alcoholics." However, a study limited to Utah and involving few respondents failed to observe the effect (Hawks, 1990; Hawks and Bahr, 1992, p. 8), as did a study marred by numerous methodological flaws and weaknesses (Bock et al., 1987, pp. 99-100; Cochran et al., 1988, pp. 263-274).

Thus, it would appear that those individuals from an abstinence environment who choose to drink are much more likely to experience problems with their drinking. Abstinence environments provide proscriptive norms regarding drinking. Such norms (Mizruchi and Perrucci (1962, pp. 393, 396; 1967, pp. 268-270) direct people "to avoid, abstain, desist and reject all forms of behavior" associated with drinking. On the other hand, prescriptive norms direct people "to act in a particular way, spelling out the forms of behavior to which the group members must conform." An example would be the directives associated with the consumption of alcoholic beverages among Orthodox Jews. In explicating the nature of proscriptive and prescriptive norms, Mizruchi and Perrucci (1967, p. 261) pointed out, "The former provides only a goal viewed negatively; the latter provides a goal viewed positively, as well as a set of means for its attainment."

It appears that highly prescriptive norms are less likely than are highly proscriptive norms to lead to pathological behavior when deviation occurs. One reason is that prescriptive norms provide clear guidance for behavior and they do so even when they are violated. However, once deviance from proscriptive norms occurs, there are no norms or guidelines for proper behavior. To the contrary, it appears that proscriptive norms are often accompanied by negative role conceptions (Skolnick, 1957, 1958; Bouchard, 1959; Fitzpatrick, 1963; Maddox and Jennings, 1959; Knupfer, 1961, p. 22; Chafetz and Demone, 1962, p. 96).

Skolnick found this in his analysis of abstinence Sunday school literature. Children were taught in that curricular material that they must not drink and that drinking is a violation of good Christian behavior because it results in problem behaviors. The literature warned of the evils of even social drinking. "Moderation is a snare put forth by liquor interests to entrap the young. If a person drinks, he will lose health, fortune and friends" (Skolnick, 1958, pp. 455-456). In this view, "drinker" is a bad word and is inextricably associated with rowdy bars, broken homes and delirium tremors (Bacon and Jones, 1968, p. 3). As Skolnick explained, "The abstinence norm appears to have two sides: on one, it promotes an attitude of repugnance toward drinking and insobriety; on the other, it associates even nominal use of beverage alcohol with insobriety and concomitant problem behaviors. Consequently, even though the idea of drinking is rejected, insobriety tends to be established as the norm *for* drinking" (1957, p. 4, emphasis his). In an abstinence environment, "the roles of drinkers are clearly defined; they either abstain or they drink to excess" (Chafetz and Demone, 1962, p. 96). Thus, individuals who violate abstinence norms by simply experimenting with alcohol tend to be cast inadvertently into playing the negative role they have been led to believe characterizes drinkers. It was Thorner's (1953) view that when individuals from an abstinence group take even one drink they immediately become alcoholics in the eyes of their fellow churchgoers. Thus, the definitions and reactions of abstinence peers, while preventing drinking among most, may help create problem drinkers among those who decide to drink any amount of alcohol.

Another reason prescriptive norms are less likely to lead to extreme behavior when deviation occurs is that deviance and conformity are not so dichotomized as in proscriptive systems; therefore, deviance is not seen as so threatening in the former. Consequently, deviance from proscriptive norms tends to result in some degree of exclusion from the group. As a result, the effectiveness of group norms over the individual tends to be reduced. This is less of a problem with regard to deviance from prescriptive norms.

A third reason is based on the fact that when drinking is defined or desired for its personal effects,[19] it tends to be associated much more often with drinking problems than when it is defined for its social effects (Larsen and Abu-

Laban, 1968; Mulford and Miller, 1960). Therefore, it is important that

[t]he prescriptive normative background, presumably because of an abundance of guidelines which define appropriate drinking behavior, tends to result in an emphasis on the use of alcohol for social rather than personal reasons. The prescriptive norms evidently disapprove drinking for personal effects. . . . Considering the nonscriptive normative background, it seems that permissiveness and anomie regarding the consumption of alcoholic beverages combine to influence the development of a personal-effects definition of alcohol (Abu-Laban and Larsen, 1968, p. 41).[20]

Blacker identified the common characteristics of groups with high rates of alcoholism as:

1) high social pressure to drink;
2) inconsistent or nonexistent social sanctions against excessive drinking[21]
3) utilitarian or convivial goals in drinking;[22] and
4) ambivalent attitudes and feelings toward moderate drinking (Blacker, 1966, p. 66).

He concluded that "in any group or society in which drinking customs, values, and sanctions--together with the attitudes of all segments of the group or society --are well established, known to and agreed upon by all, consistent with the rest of the culture, and are characterized by prescriptions for moderate drinking and proscriptions against excessive drinking, the rate of alcoholism will be low" (Blacker, 1966, p. 68).

SUMMARY AND CONCLUSION

The vast panorama of human behavior clearly demonstrates that alcohol is widely used around the world and that its use is usually seen as desirable and beneficial. It is also apparent that the social or human-interactive effects as well as the emotional or affective effects of alcohol are virtually all learned.[23] Does it make us happy or sad, aggressive or passive? These have little or nothing to do with the properties of alcohol and almost everything to do with the nature of our beliefs, attitudes and norms. Thus, sociocultural factors are essential to understanding drinking behavior.

Michael Robbins (1979, p. 363) has summarized evidence regarding the relevant social and cultural factors:

In general, it has been found that irrespective of the type of beverage (e.g., fermented or distilled) or the amount consumed, when alcohol is well integrated into the sociocultural system (i.e., positively regarded as a necessary and appropriate component of a wide variety of activities and accepted from an early age), little or no emphasis is placed on its "escape-providing" qualities or psychological problem-solving, personal effects.

Instead its positive social value in facilitating convivial social interaction, its cultural value in sacred, ceremonial observances, and physiological value as a healthful enhancement of the diet will assure prime importance.

More specifically, the consumption of alcohol for personal effects will be minimized (and, hence, alcohol problems will be minimized) when drinking is

1) the prescriptive norm,
2) an important expression of social relationships, religious observances, and other customary activities,
3) learned early and in domestic settings,
4) a frequent accompaniment of meals and thought to be of nutritional and medicinal value, and
5) where consumption patterns are regulated and controlled by custom in a known, agreed upon, and consistent manner . . . (Robbins, 1979, p. 363).

On the other hand, alcohol will be used primarily for its personal effects (and, hence, tend to be more often associated with drinking problems) when it

1) is a source of social and emotional concern,
2) occurs in an ambivalent or nonscriptive normative environment.
3) has been recently introduced [to the society],
4) is not interwoven with family, social, or religious institutions,
5) is not a part of meals,
6) is learned later in life,
7) occurs mainly outside of the family in secular situations,
8) is associated with status transformations from adolescence to adulthood, and
9) is thought to be a personal disinhibitor of socially undesirable sexual and aggressive behavior (and as a consequence often is; cf. MacAndrew and Edgerton, 1969) . . . (Robbins, 1979, pp. 163-164).

It should be clear that attitudes, beliefs and social norms profoundly influence the way in which people behave when they drink as well as the resulting incidence of drinking problems (or lack of problems) in their group or society. Mulford (1982, pp. 454-455) has made the important point: "Epidemiological findings, such as the lower alcoholism rates for women than for men, and the trend for the traditionally lower rural rate to catch up with the urban rate, suggests that alcohol abuse is more of a people problem involving judgments, values, and so forth, and less of a technical problem amenable to a quick fix, as the disease concept and medical model lead us to suppose." He explains, "If, as the findings to date suggest, more effective prevention lies in the development of more responsible norms and informal controls, then epidemiologists might help communities do this by identifying the drinking attitudes and practices most highly associated with responsible drinking, as well as those associated with alcohol abuse."

Societies experience the types of behavior that they permit.

NOTES

1. For a brief review of drinking motivation literature, see Rorabaugh (1979, pp. 241-246).

2. While this quotation also appears almost word for word in Robinson (1979, pp. 25-26), it was earlier published by Mandelbaum in 1965 (and reprinted in 1979). Extensive material published by Mandelbaum in 1965 appears without acknowledgment by Robinson in 1979.

3. Consumption of "coconut toddys" is often associated with disinhibited behavior on other islands as reported by many observers, including Robert Louis Stevenson, who referred to the drink as a "devilish intoxicant, the counsellor of crime" (Stevenson, 1912, vol. 18, p. 238 cited by MacAndrew and Edgerton, 1969, p. 28).

4. Other Western examples of normative factors in alcohol-related aggression are presented by Coid (1986, p. 186).

5. Also see Marlatt (1987a, 1987b).

6. National Institute on Alcohol Abuse and Alcoholism.

7. Another observer (Fumento, 1992, p. 14) in discussing AIDS statistics is more explicit about motives:

> "The motives of the government and its bureaucracy can be understood easily enough. They are the same motives that always drive government. One is the attempt to justify the existence of bureaucratic jobs and to expand bureaucratic power. The AIDS crisis is exaggerated for the same reason the folks at the Small Business Administration will tell you that but for them American small business would go the way of the dinosaur; for the same reason EPA will tell you that but for them Americans would by now have been wiped out by exposure to lead, asbestos, and dioxin."

8. Not only does alcohol cause fewer problems than often imagined in the United States, but cross-cultural analysis has identified important functions that it often performs (Gordon, 1984, pp. 357-362; Collman, 1979; Room, 1992, pp. 100 and 103). For example:

> In many ethnographic reports, heavy emphasis is laid on the socially integrative functions of alcohol. Among American Indians on Skid Row, Brody (1970) found that drinking "unites Indians as Indians"; in a similar context, bottle-sharing was similarly frequent and socially significant among white "winos" (Spradley 1970). Among the Buganda, the traditional homebrew is integral to many social relationships . . . (M. Robbins 1977). An Australian Aboriginal population use liquor effectively as a means of building social credit (Collmann 1979); so do the Papago (Waddell 1973, 1975) and the Giriama (Parkin 1972). Maize beer "is the most important thread in the loose fabric of LoBir life" (Hagaman 1980: 205), and women earn social status on the basis of their skill at making it. The importance of socialization while drinking is emphasized as providing a sense of communitas for Swiss villagers (Gibson and Weinberg 1980) . . . (Heath, 1987, pp. 31-32).

9. Alcoholism rates of the Jews are often reported to be as low as one fortieth that of the Irish, thus prompting Blume and Dropkin to begin a publication with the anonymous quote "You're going to study Jewish alcoholics? All three of them?" (cited

in Blume and Dropkin, 1980, p. 123). For a review of early anecdotal and statistical evidence, see Meystel (1949, ch. 2).

10. A continuing definition of alcoholism as being non-Jewish would appear to be an important factor contributing to the denial of alcoholism, as Spiegel (1981) and Levy (1982) have observed.

11. For extensive documentation of Irish-American insobriety, see chapter one of Stivers' (1976, pp. 1-14) book.

12. This prohibition has now been lifted by the Church.

13. Not only do Italians view wine as a healthful beverage, but some perceive it as a medication (Simboli, 1985, p. 64):

> Silone (1962) describes Cassarola, an Italian folk healer, and her wine prescription. The customer asks for assistance regarding her three-year old daughter who is suffering from some illness. Cassarola prescribes a glass of wine for the little girl every morning. The girl's mother questions the prescription by saying, "She's only three years old." Cassarola responds confidently, "She's already three? Well, then you can give her a glass of wine at night too" (p. 106).

14. "Acculturation is a process that theoretically begins when the first generation (or immigrant group) comes into first-hand continuous contact with the host society and starts changing its traditional behavior patterns to conform to the host society" (Simboli, 1985, p. 62).

15. Most residents emigrated from or were descended from four contiguous counties (*hsien*) in the province of Kwangtung, and are generally known as the "Cantonese" (Barnett, 1955, p. 180).

16. In spite of its title (which only makes reference to Native Hawaiians, Japanese, Filipinos and Caucasians), this paper presents data on the Chinese.

17. It has been hypothesized that this is caused by a sudden increase of acetaldehyde in the blood occurring when Asians drink, because they have a higher initial rate of alcohol metabolism (Kitano, 1989, p. 146). In any case, the Chinese expression "to be red faced," for being slightly intoxicated clearly has a basis in fact (Anderson and Anderson, 1977, p. 343; Anderson, 1988, p. 121).

18. Members of the Church of the Nazarene must sign a pledge of abstinence (Skolnick, 1957, p. 136) and are removed from membership if they are discovered to drink after signing the pledge (Fitzpatrick, 1963, p. 29).

19. An empirical measure (Mulford, 1982, p. 443) of personal-effects drinking involves positive responses to the following items.

Would You Say These Things about Your Drinking:
1. Drinking helps me forget I am not the kind of person I really want to be.
2. Drinking helps me get along better with other people.
3. Drinking helps me feel more satisfied with myself.
4. Drinking gives me more confidence in myself.
5. Drinking helps me overcome shyness.
6. Drinking makes me less self-conscious.

20. "Nonscriptive" is Abu-Laban and Larsen's term for an environment with few or no guidelines concerning drinking. It appears to be synonymous with Durkheim's (1951) more commonly used term of "anomic."

21. Stivers has argued that for the Irish-American of this century, the meaning of hard drinking became positive: "at first one drank heavily because one was Irish, whereas now one was Irish because one drank heavily" (1985, p. 124). He (Stivers, 1976, p. 130) contends that hard drinking acquired "all the appearance of a religious obligation--the obligation to be Irish and to promote one's Irishness. The implication was that the more one drank, the more Irish one became." Also see Stivers (1978, p. 130).

22. In these, the intention is "to promote fun and pleasure, physical states of well-being, and the gratification of self-interests such as the release of inner tensions" (Blacker, 1966, p. 63).

23. Naturally, effects on equilibrium, judgments of time and distance, rate of urination, dilation of blood vessels, etc., clearly result from the pharmacological properties of alcohol.

REFERENCES

Abu-Laban, Baha and Larsen, Donald E.   The qualities and sources of norms and definitions of alcohol. *Sociology and Social Research*, 1968, *53*, 34-43.

Ahern, Frank M. Alcohol Use and Abuse among Four Ethnic Groups in Hawaii: Native Hawaiians, Japanese, Filipinos, and Caucasians. In: Speigler, Danielle, Tate, Diane, Aitken, Sherrie, and Christian, Charles (eds.) *Alcohol Abuse among U.S. Ethnic Minorities*. Rockville, MD: National Institute on Alcohol Abuse and Alcoholism, 1985. pp. 315-328.

Akutsu, Phillip D., Sue, Stanley, Nolan, W. S. Sane, and Nakamura, Charles Y. Ethnic differences in alcohol consumption among Asians and Caucasians in the United States: An investigation of cultural and physiological factors. *Journal of Studies on Alcohol*, 1989, *50*, 261-267.

Albrecht, S. L. Alcohol Consumption and Abuse. Paper presented at Utah Academy of Arts at Sciences, Provo, UT, Brigham Young University, May 1985. Reported by Rick D. Hawks in Alcohol Use among LDS and Other Groups Teaching Abstinence. Unpublished paper, 1990.

American Psychiatric Association.   *Diagnostic and Statistical Manual of Mental Disorders*. 3rd edition. Washington, DC: American Psychiatric Association, 1980.

Anderson, Jr., Eugene N. *The Food of China*. New Haven, CT and London: Yale University Press, 1988.

Anderson, Jr., Eugene N., and Anderson Marja L. Modern China: South. In: Chang, K. C. (ed.) *Food in Chinese Culture: Anthropological and Historical Perspectives*. New Haven, CT and London: Yale University Press, 1977. pp. 317-382.

Arensberg, Conrad M., and Kimball, S. T. *Family and Community in Ireland*. Cambridge, MA: Harvard University Press, 1940.

Armor, David J., Polich, J. Michael, and Stambul, Harriet B. *Alcoholism and Treatment*. New York: John Wiley and Sons, 1978.

Armyr, Gunno, Elmer, Ake, and Herz, Ulrich. *Alcohol in the World of the 80's*. Stockholm, Sweden: Sober Forlags, 1982.

Bacon, Margaret and Jones, Mary B. *Teenage Drinking*. New York: Crowell, 1968.

Bacon, Selden D.   Studies of drinking in Jewish culture: I. General introduction. *Quarterly Journal of Studies on Alcohol*, 1951, *12*, 444-450.

Bailey, M. B., Haberman, P. W., and Alkene, H. The epidemiology of alcoholism in an urban residential area. *Quarterly Journal of Studies on Alcohol*, 1965, *26*, 19-40.

Bales, Robert F. The "Fixation Factor" in Alcohol Addiction: An Hypothesis Derived from a Comparative Study of Irish and Jewish Social Norms. Ph.D. dissertation, Harvard University, 1944. Published by Arno Press, 1980.

Bales, Robert F. Cultural differences in rates of alcoholism. *Quarterly Journal of Studies on Alcohol*, 1946, *6*, pp. 480-499.

Bales, Robert F. Attitudes toward Drinking in the Irish Culture. In: Pittman, David J. and Snyder, Charles R. (eds.) *Society, Culture, and Drinking Patterns*. New York: Wiley, 1962. pp. 157-187.

Barnett, Milton L. Alcoholism in the Cantonese of New York City: In Anthropological Study. In: Diethelm, Oskar (ed.) *Etiology of Chronic Alcoholism*. Springfield, IL: Charles C. Thomas, 1955. pp. 179-227.

Bates, Marston, and Abbott, D. D. *Coral Island: Portrait of an Atoll*. New York: Charles Scribner's Sons, 1958.

Berreman, G. Drinking patterns of the Aleuts. *Quarterly Journal of Studies on Alcohol*, 1956, *17*, 503-514.

Blacker, Edward. Sociocultural factors in alcoholism. *International Psychiatry Clinics*, 1966 *3*, pp. 51-80.

Blaine, Allan. Introduction. In: Blaine, Allan (ed.) *Alcoholism and the Jewish Community*. New York: Federation of Jewish Philanthropies of New York, 1980. pp. 7-17.

Blane, Howard T. Acculturation and drinking in an Italian American community. *Journal of Studies on Alcohol*. 1977, *38*, 1324-1346.

Blume, Sheila, and Dropkin, Dee. The Jewish Alcoholic - An Unrecognized Minority. In: Blaine, Allan (ed.) *Alcoholism and the Jewish Community*. New York: Federation of Jewish Philanthropies of New York, 1980. pp. 123-134.

Bock, E. Wilbur, Cochran, John K. and Beeghley, Leonard. Moral messages: The relative influence of denomination on the religiosity-alcohol relationship. *Sociological Quarterly*, 1987, *28*, 89-103.

Bonavia, David. *The Chinese*. New York: Lippincott & Crowell, 1980.

Bouchard, P. L. Parent-Child Relationships and Alcoholism: A Case Study of the Histories of Sixty-Eight Alcoholics to Determine the Effect of Early Developmental Factors on the Acceptance of Parental Teachings about Drinking. Unpublished master's thesis. University of Toronto, 1959.

Brandes, S. Drinking patterns and alcohol control in a Castilian mountain village. *Anthropology*, 1979, *3*, 1-15.

Brody, Hugh. *Indians on Skid Row*. Ottawa: Northern Science Research Group, Department of Indian Affairs and Northern Development Publication, 1970.

Brody, Hugh. *Innishkillane: Change and Decline in the West of Ireland*. London: Allen Lane, Penguin Press, 1973.

Brown, H. B. *Mormonism*. Salt Lake City, UT: Deseret News Press, 1963.

Bunzel, Ruth. The role of alcohol in two Central American cultures. *Psychiatry*, 1940, *3*, 361-387.

Burrows, E. G. From value to ethos on Ifaluk atoll. *Southwestern Journal of Anthropology*, 1952, *8*, 13-35.

Burrows, E. G., and Spiro, Milford E. *An Atoll Culture: Ethnography of Ifaluk in the Central Carolines*. New Haven, CT: Human Relations Area Files, 1953.

Cahalan, Don. *Problem Drinkers*. San Francisco: Jossey-Bass, 1970.

Cahalan, Don and Room, Robin. *Problem Drinking among American Men*. New Brunswick, NJ: Rutgers Center for Alcohol Studies, 1974. Research monograph No. 7.

Cahalan, Don. Why does the alcoholism field act like a ship of fools? *British Journal of Addiction*, 1979, *74*, 235-238.

Cahalan, Don. *Understanding America's Drinking Problem*. San Francisco, CA: Jossey-Bass, 1987.

Carstairs, G. M. Daru and Bhang: Cultural Factors in the Choice of Intoxicant. In: Marshall, Mac (ed.) *Beliefs, Behaviors, & Alcoholic Beverages: A Cross-Cultural Survey*. Ann Arbor, MI: University of Michigan Press, 1979. pp. 297-312. Originally published in *Quarterly Journal of Studies on Alcohol*, 1954, *15*, 220-237.

Chafetz, Morris. Consumption of alcohol in the Far and Middle East. *The New England Journal of Medicine*, 1964, *217*, 297-301.

Chafetz, Morris E., and Demone, Harold W., Jr. *Alcoholism and Society*. New York: Oxford University Press, 1962.

Chauncey, Robert L. New careers for moral entrepreneurs: Teenage drinking. *Journal of Drug Issues*, 1980, 45-70.

Cheinisse, L. La race Juive jouit-elle d'une immunité à l'égard de l'alcoolisme? *La Semaine Médicale*, 1908, *28*, 613-615. Cited by Snyder, Charles R., Palgi, Eldar, Pnina, and Elian, Beatrice. Alcoholism among the Jews in Israel: A pilot study. I. Research rationale and a look at the ethnic factor. *Journal of Studies on Alcohol*. 1982, *43*, 623-654. p. 624.

Chi, Iris, Kitano, Harry H. L., and Lubben, James E. Male Chinese drinking behavior in Los Angeles. *Journal of Studies on Alcohol*, 1988, *49*, 21-25.

Chi, Iris, Lubben, James E., and Kitano, Harry H. L. Differences in drinking behavior among three Asian-American groups. *Journal of Studies on Alcohol*, 1989, *50*, 15-23.

Chu, G. Drinking patterns and attitudes of rooming-house Chinese in San Francisco. *Quarterly Journal of Studies on Alcohol*, Supplement, 1972, *6*.

Cochran, John D., Beeghley, Leonard, and Bock, E. Wilbur. Religiosity and alcohol behavior: An exploration of reference group theory. *Sociological Forum*, 1988, *3*, 256-276.

Coid, Jeremy. Socio-Cultural Factors in Alcohol-Related Aggression. In: Brian, Paul F. (ed.) *Alcohol and Aggression*. London, England: Croom Helm, 1986. pp. 184-211.

Collmann, Jeff. Social order and the exchange of liquor: A theory of drinking among Australian Aborigines. *Journal of Anthropological Research*, 1979, *35*, 208-224.

Culver, Ronald E. Cultural and Ethnic Comparisons of Alcohol Use and the Effect of Acculturation on the Drinking Behavior of American Immigrants. Unpublished M.L.S. thesis, University of Toledo, 1987.

Davies, J., and Stacey, B. *Teenagers and Alcohol. Vol. 2. An Enquiry Carried Out on Behalf of the Health Education Unit of the Scottish Home and Health Department*. London: HMSO, 1972.

de la Fontaine, Elise. Cultural and Psychological Implications in Case Work Treatment with Irish Clients. In: Family Welfare Association of America. *Cultural Problems in Social Case Work*. New York: Family Welfare Association of America, 1940.

Dobrizhoffer, Martin. *An Account of the Abipones, an Equestrian People of Paraguay*. Vol. 3. London: John Murray, 1822.

Durkheim, Emile. *Suicide.* New York: Free Press, 1951.

Fein, L. G. Religious observance and mental health: A note. *The Journal of Pastoral Care*, 1958, *12*, 99-101.

Fitzpatrick, Laura E. J. The Relation between Religious Beliefs and the Use of Beverage Alcohol. Unpublished master's thesis, University of Toronto, 1963.

Ford, Gene. *The Benefits of Moderate Drinking: Alcohol, Health, and Society.* San Francisco: Wine Appreciation Guild, 1988.

Ford, J. C. *What About Your Drinking?* New York: Paulist Press, 1961.

Fumento, Michael. Teenage AIDS and anal ideologues. *Heterodoxy*, 1992, *1*, 1 & 14.

Garvin, W. C. Post-Prohibition alcoholic psychoses in New York State. *American Journal of Psychiatry*, 1930, *86*, 739-754.

Gibson, James A., and Weinberg, Daniela. In *vino communitas*: Wine and identity in a Swiss Alpine village. *Anthropological Quarterly*, 1980, *52*, 111-121.

Glad, Donald D. Attitudes and experiences of American-Jewish and American-Irish male youth as related to differences in adult rates of inebriety. *Quarterly Journal of Studies on Alcohol*, 1947, *8*, 406-472.

Glad, Donald D. Attitude and Experience of American-Jewish and American-Irish Male Youth as Related to Differences in Rates of Inebriety. Unpublished Ph.D. dissertation, Stanford University, 1947.

Glassner, Barry and Berg, Bruce. Jewish-Americans and Alcohol: Processes of Avoidance and Definition. In: Bennett, Linda A. and Ames, Genevieve M. (eds.) *The American Experience with Alcohol: Contrasting Cultural Perspectives.* New York: Plenum, 1985. pp. 93-107.

Glatt, M. M. Alcoholism and Drug Dependence Amongst Jews. In: Blaine, Allan (ed.) *Alcoholism and the Jewish Community.* New York: Federation of Jewish Philanthropies of New York, 1980. pp. 187-201. Originally published in *British Journal of Addiction*, 1970, *64*, 297-304.

Globetti, Gerald. Prohibition Norms and Teenage Drinking. In: Ewing, J. A., and Rouse, Beatrice A. (eds.) *Drinking Alcohol in American Society - Issues and Current Research.* Chicago: Nelson-Hall, Inc., 1978. pp. 159-170.

Gordon, Andrew J. Alcohol Use in the Perspective of Cultural Anthropology. In: Galanter, Marc (ed.) *Recent Developments in Alcoholism*, Volume 2. New York: Plenum Press, 1984. pp. 355-375.

Gorer, Geoffrey. *Himalayan Village: An Account of the Lepchas of Sikkim.* London: Michael Joseph Ltd., 1938.

Greeley, Andrew M., and McCready, William C. The Transmission of Cultural Heritage: The Case of the Irish and the Italians. In: Glazer, Nathan, and Moynihan, Daniel P. (eds.) *Ethnicity and Experience.* Cambridge, MA: Harvard University Press, 1975. pp. 209-235.

Greeley, Andrew M., McCready, William C., and Theisen, Gary. *Ethnic Drinking Subcultures.* New York: Praeger, 1980.

Gross, Leonard. *How Much Is too Much: The Effects of Social Drinking.* New York: Random House, 1983.

Gusfield, Joseph. *The Culture of Public Problems.* Chicago, IL: University of Chicago Press, 1981.

Hagaman, Barbara L. Food for thought: Beer in a social and ritual context in a West African Society. *Journal of Drug Issues*, 1980, *10*, 203-214.

Haggard, H. W., and Jellinek, E. M. *Alcohol Explored.* New York: Doubleday, 1942.

Hamer, J. H.   Acculturation Stress and the Functions of Alcohol among the Forest Potawatomi. In: Hamer, J. H., and Steinbring, J. (eds.) *Alcohol and Native Peoples of the North.* Lanham, MD: University Press of America, 1980.

Hanson, David J. Norm Qualities and Deviant Drinking Behavior. Unpublished Ph.D. dissertation, Syracuse University, 1972.

Hanson, David J. Drinking norms and aggression. *Psychology,* 1978, *15*, 34.

Hawks, Ricky D. Alcohol Use among LDS and other Groups Teaching Abstinence. In: Watson, R. R. (ed.) *Drugs and Alcohol Abuse Prevention.* Clifton, NJ: The Humana Press, 1990. pp. 133-149.

Hawks, Ricky D. and Bahr, Stephen H. Religion and drug use. *Journal of Drug Education,* 1992, *22*, 1-8.

Heath, Dwight B. Drinking patterns of the Bolivian Camba. *Quarterly Journal of Studies on Alcohol,* 1958, *19*, 491-508.

Heath, Dwight B. Drinking patterns of the Bolivian Camba. In: Pittman, David J. and Snyder, Charles R. (eds.) *Society, Culture, and Drinking Patterns.* New York: John Wiley and Sons, 1962. pp. 22-36. Revision of article of same title, *Quarterly Journal of Studies on Alcohol,* 1958, *19*, 491-508.

Heath, Dwight B. A Decade of Development in the Anthropological Study of Alcohol Use: 1970-1980. In: Douglas, Mary (ed.) *Constructive Drinking: Perspectives on Drink from Anthropology.* Cambridge, England: Cambridge University Press, 1987. pp. 16-69.

Heien, Dale M., and Pittman, David J. The economic costs of alcohol abuse: An assessment of current methods and estimates. *Journal of Studies on Alcohol,* 1989, *50*, 567-579.

Helzer, J. E., Canino, G. J., Yeh, E. K., Bland, R. C., Lee, C. K., Hwu, H. G., and Newman, S. Alcoholism - North America and Asia. *Archives of General Psychiatry,* 1990, *47*, 313-319.

Henry, Jules. *Jungle People: A Kaingáng Tribe of the Highlands of Brazil.* Richmond, VA: J. J. Augustin, 1941.

Heok, K. E. Drinking habits of elderly Chinese. *British Journal of Addiction,* 1990, *85*, 571-573.

Hogan, Edmond P. Religious Affiliation, Norm Quality, and Drinking Patterns of Adolescents. Unpublished Ph.D. dissertation, Washington State University, 1979.

Honigmann, John J. Dynamics of Drinking in an Austrian Village. In: Marshall, Mac (ed.) *Beliefs, Behaviors, & Alcoholic Beverages: A Cross-Cultural Survey.* Ann Arbor, MI: University of Michigan Press, 1979. pp. 414-428. Originally published in *Ethnology,* 1963, *2*, 157-169.

Hsu, Francis L. K. *Americans and Chinese.* New York: Natural History Press, 1970.

Hunter, Monica. Reacting to Conquest: Effects of Contact with Europeans of the Pondo of South Africa. London: Oxford University Press, 1961.

Hurt, W. R., and Brown, R. M. Social drinking patterns of the Yankton Sioux. *Human Organization,* 1965, *24*, 222-230.

Hutchinson, Bertram. Alcohol as a Contributing Factor in Social Disorganization: The South African Bantu in the Nineteenth Century. In: Marshall, Mac (ed.) *Beliefs, Behaviors, & Alcoholic Beverages: A Cross-Cultural Survey.* Ann Arbor, MI: University of Michigan Press, 1979. pp. 328-341. Originally published in *Revista de Anthropologia,* 1961, *9*.

Hyde, R. W., and Chisholm, R. Studies in medical sociology: III. The relation of mental disorders to race and nationality. *New England Journal of Medicine*, 1944, *231*, 612-618.

Isralowitz, Richard, and Hong, Ong Teck. Singapore: A study of university students' drinking behavior. *British Journal of Addiction*, 1988, *83*, 1321-1323.

Jellinek, E. Morton. A document on the reformation period of inebriety: Sebastian Franck's 'On the Horrible Vice of Drunkenness,' etc. *Quarterly Journal of Studies on Alcohol*, 1941a, *2*, 391-395.

Jellinek, E. Morton. Immanuel Kant on Drinking. *Quarterly Journal of Studies on Alcohol*, 1941b, *1*, 777-778.

Jellinek, E. Morton. Estimate of Number of Alcoholics and Rates of Alcoholics per 100,000 Adult Population (20 Years and Older) for Certain Countries. In: Expert Committee on Mental Health. *Report on the First Session of the Alcoholism Subcommittee*. Geneva: World Health Organization, 1951 (Technical Report Series, No. 42). Annex I. pp. 19-20.

Jellinek, E. Morton. Cultural Differences in the Meaning of Alcohol. In: Pittman, David J., and Snyder, Charles R. (eds.) *Society, Culture, and Drinking Patterns*. New York: John Wiley & Sons, 1962. pp. 382-388.

Jessor, Richard, Young H. B., Young, E. B., and Tesi, G. Perceived opportunity, alienation and drinking behavior among Italian and American youth. *Journal of Personality and Social Psychology*, 1970, *15*, 215-222.

Jones, Evan. Student Drinking in the High Schools of Utah. Unpublished masters thesis, University of Utah, 1957.

Jones, Howard. *Alcoholic Addiction: A Psycho-Social Approach to Abnormal Drinking*. London: Tavistock, 1963.

Josephson, E. An Assessment of Statistics on Alcohol-Related Problems, Trends in Problem Drinking. Columbia University School of Public Health. Distilled Spirits Council of the United States, May 5, 1980. Quoted in Ford, Gene. *The Benefits of Moderate Drinking*. San Francisco: Wine Appreciation Guild, 1988, p. 135.

Junod, Henri A. *The Life of a South African Tribe*. Vol. I. London: Macmillan and Co., 1927.

Keller, Mark. Introduction. In: Lolli, Giorgio, Serianni, Emidio, Golder, Grace M., and Luzzatto-Fegiz, Pierpaolo. *Alcohol in Italian Culture*. Glencoe, IL: Free Press, 1958. pp. xi-xv.

Keller, Mark. The Great Jewish Drink Mystery. In: Marshall, Mac (ed.) *Beliefs, Behaviors & Alcoholic Beverages: A Cross-Cultural Survey*. Ann Arbor, MI: University of Michigan Press, 1979. pp. 404-414. Originally published in *British Journal of Addiction*, 1970, *64*, 287-296.

Kennedy, John G. *Tarahumara of the Sierra Madra: Beer, Ecology and Social Organization*. Arlington Heights, IL: AHM Publishing, 1978.

Kennedy, R. *The Irish*. Berkeley, CA: University of California Press, 1973.

King, A. R. The alcohol problem in Israel. *Quarterly Journal of Studies on Alcohol*, 1961, *22*, 321-324.

Kitano, Harry H. L. Alcohol and the Asian American. In: Watts, Thomas D. and Wright, Roosevelt, Jr. (eds.) *Alcoholism in Minority Populations*. Springfield, IL: Charles C. Thomas, 1989. pp. 143-156.

Kitano, Harry H. L. and Chi, Iris. Asian Americans and Alcohol: The Chinese, Japanese, Koreans, and Filipinos in Los Angeles. In: Spiegler, Danielle, Tate, Diane, Aiken, Sherrie, and Christian, Charles (eds.) *Alcohol Abuse among U.S. Ethnic Minorities*.

Rockville, MD: National Institute on Alcohol Abuse and Alcoholism, 1985. pp. 373-382.

Knupfer, Genevieve. *California Drinking Practices Study No. 3, Characteristics of Abstainers*. Berkeley, CA: State of California Department of Public Health, 1961.

Knupfer, Genevieve, and Room, Robin. Drinking patterns and attitudes of Irish, Jewish and White Protestant American men. *Quarterly Journal of Studies on Alcohol*, 1967, *28*, 676-699.

Kupferer, H. J. A case of sanctioned drinking: The Rupert's House Cree. *Anthropological Quarterly*, 1979, *52*, 198-203.

LaBarre, Weston. Some observations on character structure in the Orient. II. The Chinese. Part Two. *Psychiatry*, 1946, *9*, 375-395.

Landman, R. H. Studies of drinking in Jewish culture. III. Drinking patterns of children and adolescents attending religious schools. *Quarterly Journal of Studies on Alcohol*, 1952, *13*, 87-94.

Larsen, Donald E., and Abu-Laban, Baha. Norm qualities and deviant drinking behavior. *Social Problems*, 1968, *15*, 441-450.

Lawrence, Joseph J. and Maxwell, Milton A. Drinking and Socio-Economic Status. In: Pittman, David J. and Snyder, Charles R. (eds.) *Society, Culture, and Drinking Patterns*. New York: John Wiley & Sons, 1962. pp. 141-145.

LeMarchand, Loic, Kolonel, Laurence N., and Yoshizawa, Carl N. Alcohol Consumption Patterns among the Five Major Ethnic Groups in Hawaii: Correlations with the Incidence of Esophageal and Oropharyngeal Cancer. In: Spiegler, Danielle, Tate, Diane, Aitken, Sherrie and Christian, Charles (eds.) *Alcohol Abuse among U.S. Ethnic Minorities*. Rockville, MD: National Institute on Alcohol Abuse and Alcoholism, 1985. pp. 355-371.

Lemert, Edwin M. Forms and Pathology of Drinking in Three Polynesian Societies. In: Marshall, Mac (ed.) *Beliefs, Behaviors, & Alcoholic Beverages: A Cross-Cultural Survey*. Ann Arbor, MI: University of Michigan Press, 1979. pp. 192-208. Originally published in *American Anthropologist*, 1964, *66*, 361-374.

Levy, J. E., and Kunitz, S. J. *Indian Drinking: Navajo Practices and Anglo-American Theories*. New York: John Wiley & Sons, 1974.

Levy, S. J. Dealing with denial: Alcoholism among Jews. *Bulletin of the Society for the Psychology of Substance Abuse, 1982, 1*, 55-58.

Lin, T. Y. A study of the incidence of mental disorder in Chinese and other cultures. *Psychiatry*, 1953, *16*, 313-336.

Linsky, Arnold S., Colby, Jr., John P., and Straus, Murray A. Drinking norms and alcohol-related problems in the United States. *Journal of Studies on Alcohol*, 1986, *47*, 384-393.

Lisansky, E. S., Golder, Grace, and Lolli, Giorgio. Relationship of personality adjustment to eating and drinking patterns in a group of Italian Americans. *Quarterly Journal of Studies on Alcohol*. 1954, *15*, 545-561.

Lolli, Giorgio, Serianni, Emidio, Golder, Grace M., and Luzzatto-Fegiz, Pierpeolo. *Alcohol in Italian Culture: Food and Wine in Relation to Sobriety among Italians and Italian Americans*. Glencoe, IL: Free Press, 1958.

Lurie, Nancy O. The World's Oldest On-Going Protest Demonstration: North American Indian Drinking Patterns. In: Marshall, Mac (ed.) *Beliefs, Behaviors & Alcoholic Beverages: A Cross-Cultural Survey*. Ann Arbor, MI: University of Michigan Press, 1979. pp. 127-145. Originally published in *Pacific Historical Review*, 1971, *40*, 311-

332.

MacAndrew, Craig, and Edgerton, Robert. *Drunken Comportment: A Social Explanation.* Chicago, IL: Aldine, 1969.

Maddox, George L. Teenage Drinking in the United States. In: Pittman, David J. and Snyder, Charles R. (eds.) *Society, Culture, and Drinking Patterns.* New York: John Wiley & Sons, 1962. pp. 230-245.

Maddox, George L., and Jennings, Audrey, M. An analysis of fantasy: an exploratory study of social definitions of alcohol and its use by means of a projective technique. *Quarterly Journal of Studies on Alcohol,* 1959, *20,* 334-345.

Maddox, George L., and McCall, Bevode L. *Drinking among Teen-Agers.* New Brunswick, NJ: Rutgers Center of Alcohol Studies, 1964.

Mäkelä, Klaus. Level of Consumption and Social Consequences of Drinking. In: Israel, Yedy, Glaser, Frederik B., Kalant, Harold, Popham, Robert E., Schmidt, Wolfgang and Smart, Reginald G. (eds.) *Research Advances in Alcohol and Drug Problems.* Vol. 4. New York: Plenum, 1978. pp. 303-348.

Mandelbaum, David G. Alcohol and Culture. In: Marshall, Mac (ed.) *Beliefs, Behaviors, & Alcoholic Beverages: A Cross-Cultural Survey.* Ann Arbor, MI: University of Michigan Press, 1979. pp. 14-30. Originally published in *Current Anthropology,* 1965, *6,* 281-293.

Mangin, William. Drinking among Andean Indians. *Quarterly Journal of Studies on Alcohol,* 1957, *18,* 55-66.

Marciniak, Marek L. Filters, Strainers and Siphons in Wine and Beer Production and Drinking Customs in Ancient Egypt. Paper presented at Annual Alcohol Epidemiology Symposium of the Kettil Bruun Society for Social and Epidemiological Research on Alcohol. Toronto, Ontario: May 30-June 5, 1992.

Marlatt, G. Alan. Alcohol, expectancy, and emotional states: How drinking patterns may be affected by beliefs about alcohol's effects. *Alcohol Health and Research World,* 1987a, *11,* 10-13, 80-81.

Marlatt, G. Alan. Alcohol, the Magic Elixir: Stress, Expectancy, and the Transformation of Emotional States. In: Gottheil, E., Druley, K. A., Pashko, S. and Weinstein, S. P. (eds.) *Stress and Addiction.* New York: Brunner/Mazel, 1987b.

Marlatt, G. Alan and Rohsenow, Damaris J. The think-drink effect. *Psychology Today,* 1981, *15,* 60-69, 93.

Marshall, Donald S. *Cuna Folk: A Conceptual Scheme Involving the Dynamic Factors of Culture as Applied to the Cuna Indians at Darien.* Unpublished Ph.D. dissertation, Harvard University, 1950.

Marshall, Mac. Conclusions. In: Marshall, Mac (ed.) *Beliefs, Behaviors, & Alcoholic Beverages: A Cross-Cultural Survey.* Ann Arbor, MI: University of Michigan Press, 1979. pp. 451-457.

Marshall, Mac. *Weekend Warriors: Alcohol in a Micronesian Culture.* Palo Alto, CA: Mayfield, 1979a.

Marshall, Mac. "Four Hundred Rabbits": An Anthropological View of Ethanol as a Disinhibitor. In: Room, Robin, and Collins, Gary (eds.) *Alcohol and Disinhibition: Nature and Meaning of the Link.* Rockville, MD: National Institute on Alcohol Abuse and Alcoholism, 1981. pp. 186-204.

Mauss, Armand L. Science, Social Movements, and Cynicism: Appreciating the Political Context of Sociological Research in Alcohol Studies. In: Roman, Paul M. (ed.) *Alcohol: The Development of Sociological Perspectives on Use and Abuse.*

New Brunswick, NJ: Rutgers Center of Alcohol Studies, 1991. pp. 187-204.

McGoldrick, M. Irish Families. In: McGoldrick, M., Pearce, J. K. and Giordano, J. (eds.) *Ethnicity and Family Therapy*, New York: Guilford Press, 1982. pp. 310-339.

Medical Gazette. Mental health in Singapore, 1987, p. 88. Cited by Isralowitz, Richard and Hong, Ang Teck. Singapore: A study of university students' drinking behavior. *British Journal of Addiction*, 1988, *83*, 1321-1323.

Meystel, Isadore. The Social Factor Accounting for the Low Incidence of Insobriety in the Jewish Community. Unpublished M.A. thesis, University of Chicago, 1949.

Mizruchi, Ephraim H., and Perrucci, Robert. Norm qualities and differential effects of deviant behavior: an exploratory analysis. *American Sociological Review*, 1962, *27*, 391-399.

Mizruchi, Ephraim H., and Perrucci, Robert. Norm Qualities and Deviant Behavior. In: Mizruchi, Ephraim H. (ed.) *The Substance of Sociology*. New York: Appleton-Century-Crofts, 1967.

Mohatt, Gerald. The Sacred Water: The Quest for Personal Power through Drinking among the Teton Sioux. In: McClelland, David C., Davis, William N., Kalin, Rudolf and Wanner, Eric (eds.) *The Drinking Man*. New York: Free Press, 1972. pp. 261-275.

Morgan, Patricia. Notes on the Italian alcohol experience. *The Drinking and Drug Practices Surveyor*, 1982, No. 18, 15-17.

Moros, N. The alcoholic personality. A statistical study. *Quarterly Journal of Studies on Alcohol*, 1942, *3*, 45-49.

Morris, John. *Living with the Lepchas: A Book about the Sikkim Himalayas*. London: William Heinemann, 1938.

Moss, F. E. and Janzen, F. V. *Types of Drinkers in Indian Communities*. Salt Lake City, UT: University of Utah, Western Region Alcoholism Training Center, 1980.

Moss, L. W., and Cappannari, S.C. Folklore and medicine in an Italian village. *Journal of American Folklore*, 1960, *73*, 95-102.

Moss, L., and Thompson, W. H. The south Italian family: Literature and observation. *Human Organization*, 1959, *18*, 35-41.

Muhlin, Gregory L. Ethnic differences in alcohol misuse: A striking reaffirmation. *Journal of Studies on Alcohol*, 1985, *46*, 172-173.

Mulford, Harold A. The Epidemiology of Alcoholism and Its Implications. In: Pattison, E. Mansell and Kaufman, Edward (ed.) *Encyclopedic Handbook of Alcoholism*. New York: Gardner Press, 1982. pp. 441-457.

Mulford, Harold A., and Miller, D. W. Drinking in Iowa. Part 3. A scale of definitions of alcohol related to drinking behavior. *Quarterly Journal of Studies on Alcohol*, 1960, *21*, 267-278.

Nason, James D. Sardines and Other Fried Fish: The Consumption of Alcoholic Beverages on a Micronesian Island. In: Marshall, Mac (ed.) *Beliefs, Behaviors, & Alcoholic Beverages: A Cross-Cultural Survey*. Ann Arbor, MI: University of Chicago Press, 1979. pp. 237-251. Originally published in *Journal of Studies on Alcohol*, 1975, *36*, 611-625.

Netting, Robert McC. Beer as a Locus Value among the West African Kofyar. In: Marshall, Mac (ed.) *Beliefs, Behaviors and Alcoholic Beverages: A Cross-Cultural Survey*. Ann Arbor, MI: University of Michigan Press, 1979. pp. 351-362. Originally published in *American Anthropologist*, 1964, *66*, 375-384.

New York State Bureau of Drug Addiction: All about Alcohol. In: Blaine, Allan (ed.).

Alcoholism and the Jewish Community. New York: Federation of Jewish Philanthropies of New York, 1980. pp. 17-46.

Nimuendajú, Curt. Tribes of the Lower and Middle Xingú River. In: Steward, Julian H. (ed.) *Handbook of South American Indians*. Vol. 3. *The Tropical Rain Forest Tribes*. Washington, D. C.: U.S. Government Printing Office, 1948. pp. 213-243.

Norbeck, Edward. *Takashima: A Japanese Fishing Community*. Salt Lake City, UT: University of Utah Press, 1954.

Pai, Szu M. Smoking and Alcohol Consumption Behaviors in Chinese Graduate Students and American Students: A Comparative Study. Unpublished M.S. thesis, State University of New York at Binghamton, 1991.

Parkin, David J. *Palms, Wine, and Witness: Public Spirit and Private Gain in an African Farming Community*. San Francisco, CA: Chandler, 1972.

Patai, Raphael. From 'Journey Into the Jewish Mind' - Alcoholism. In: Blaine, Allan (ed.) *Alcoholism and the Jewish Community*. New York: Federation of Jewish Philanthropies of New York, 1980. pp. 61-87.

Pittman, David J. Interview in Ford, Gene. *The Benefits of Moderate Drinking*. San Francisco, CA: Wine Appreciation Guild, 1988, p. 134.

Preston, J. D. Religiosity and adolescent drinking behavior. *The Sociological Quarterly*, 1969, *10*, 372-383.

Pullman, D. Some social correlates of attitudes toward the use of alcoholic beverages. *Quarterly Journal of Studies on Alcohol*, 1958, *19*, 623-635.

Reichel-Dolmatoff, Gerardo, and Reichel-Dolmatoff, Alicia. *The People of Aritama*. London: Routledge and Kegan Paul, 1961.

Rice, Dorothy P. The economic cost of alcohol abuse and alcohol dependence: 1990. *Alcohol Health & Research World*, 1993, *17*, 10-11.

Riley, J., Jr., and Marden, C. F. The social pattern of alcoholic drinking. *Quarterly Journal of Studies on Alcohol*, 1947, *8*, 265-273.

Ritchie, James E. *The Making of a Maori: A Case Study of a Changing Community*. Wellington, New Zealand: A. H. & A. W. Reed, 1963.

Robbins, Michael C. Problem-Drinking and the Integration of Alcohol in Rural Buganda. In: Marshall, Mac (ed.) *Beliefs, Behaviors, & Alcoholic Beverages: A Cross-Cultural Survey*. Ann Arbor, MI: University of Michigan Press, 1979. pp. 362-379. Originally published in *Medical Anthropology*, 1977, *1*.

Robbins, Michael C. Problem-drinking and the integration of alcohol in rural Buganda. *Medical Anthropology*, 1977, *1*, 1-24.

Robinson, David. Drinking Behaviour. In: Grant, Marcus, and Gwinner, Paul (ed.) *Alcoholism in Perspective*. Baltimore, MD: University Park Press, 1979. pp. 23-33.

Romney, Kimball, and Romney, Romaine. The Mixtecans of Juxtlahuaca, Mexico. In: Whiting, B. B. (ed.) *Six Cultures: Studies of Child Rearing*. New York: John Wiley and Sons, 1963. pp. 544-691.

Room, Robin. Cultural contingencies of alcoholism. *Journal of Health and Social Behavior*, 1968, *9*, 99-113.

Room, Robin. Drinking in the Rural South: Some Comparisons in a National Sample. In: Ewing, John A. and Rouse, Beatrice (eds.) *Law and Drinking Behavior*. Chapel Hill, NC: University of North Carolina, Center for Alcohol Studies, 1971. pp. 29-108.

Room, Robin. Region and Urbanization as Factors in Drinking Practices and Problems. In: Kissin, Benjamin and Begleiter, Henri (eds.) *The Pathogenesis of Alcoholism:*

Psychosocial Factors. New York: Plenum, 1983. pp. 555-604.

Room, Robin. Alcohol and ethnography: A case of "problem deflation"? *Current Anthropology*, 1984, *25*, 169-191.

Room, Robin. The impossible dream?--Routes to reducing alcohol problems in a temperate culture. *Journal of Substance Abuse*, 1992, *4*, 91-106.

Rorabaugh, William J. *The Alcoholic Republic*. New York: Oxford University Press, 1979.

Ross, H. Lawrence, and Hughes, Graham. Getting MADD in vain: drunk driving - what not to do. *The Nation*, 1986, *243*, 663-664.

Royce, James E. Sin or Solace? Religious views on alcohol and alcoholism. In: Watts, Thomas D. (ed.) *Social Thought on Alcoholism*. Malabar, FL: Robert E. Krieger Publishing Co., 1986. pp. 53-66.

Salvatore, Santo. *Intergenerational Shifts in Drinking Patterns, Opinions, Behaviors, and Personality Traits of Italian Americans*. Providence, RI: (Working Papers on Alcohol and Human Behavior, Number 6). Brown University, Department of Anthropology, 1979.

Samuelson, James. *The History of Drink*. London: Trubner and Co., 1878.

Sargent, Margaret J. Changes in Japanese Drinking Patterns. In: Marshall, Mac (ed.) *Beliefs, Behaviors, & Alcoholic Beverages: A Cross-Cultural Survey*. Ann Arbor, MI: University of Michigan Press, 1979. pp. 278-288. Originally published in *Quarterly Journal of Studies on Alcohol*, 1967, *28*, 709-722.

Savishinsky, J. S. A thematic analysis of drinking behavior in a Hare Indian community. *Papers in Anthropology*, 1977, *18*, 43-59.

Schaefer, James M. Alcohol and drugs in China - Report of a visit. *The Drinking and Drug Practices Surveyor*, 1980, No. 16, 19.

Scheper-Hughes, Nancy. *Saints, Scholars, and Schizophrenics: Mental Illness in Rural Ireland*. Berkeley, CA: University of California Press, 1970.

Schmidt, Wolfgang and Popham, Robert E. Impressions of Jewish Alcoholics. In: Blaine, Allan (ed.) *Alcoholism and the Jewish Community*. New York: Federation of Jewish Philanthropies of New York, 1980. pp. 153-166. Originally published in *Journal of Studies on Alcohol*, 1976, *37*, 931-939.

Schwartz, Theodore and Romanucci-Ross, Lola. Drinking and Inebriate Behavior in the Admiralty Islands, Melanesia. In: Marshall, Mac (ed.) *Beliefs, Behaviors, & Alcoholic Beverages: A Cross-Cultural Survey*. Ann Arbor, MI: University of Michigan Press, 1979. pp. 252-267. Originally published in *Ethos*, 1974, *2*, 153-174.

Seifert, Anne M. Religious Affiliation and Belief in the Epidemiology of Problem Drinking. Unpublished Ph.D. dissertation. University of California, Berkeley, 1972.

Shalloo, J. F. Some cultural factors in the etiology of alcoholism. *Quarterly Journal of Studies on Alcohol*, 1941, *2*, 464-478.

Silone, I. *Bread and Wine*. New York: Atheneum, 1962.

Simboli, Ben James. Acculturated Italian-American Drinking Practices. In: Bennett, Linda A., and Ames, Genevieve, M. (eds.) *The American Experience with Alcohol*. New York: Plenum Press, 1985. pp. 61-76.

Singer, K. Drinking patterns and alcoholism in the Chinese. *British Journal of Addiction*, 1972, *67*, 3-14.

Singer, K. The choice of intoxicant among the Chinese. In: Marshall, Mac (ed.) *Beliefs, Behaviors, & Alcoholic Beverages: A Cross-Cultural Survey*. Ann Arbor, MI: University of Michigan Press, 1979. pp. 313-326. Originally published in *British*

Journal of Addiction, 1974, *69*, 257-268.

Singh, Gurmeet. Comment on "The Single Distribution Theory of Alcohol Consumption." *Journal of Studies on Alcohol*, 1979, *40*, 522-524.

Skolnick, Jerome H. A study of the relation of ethnic background to arrests for inebriety. *Quarterly Journal of Studies on Alcohol*, 1954, *15*, 622-630.

Skolnick, Jerome H. The Stumbling Block: A Sociological Study of the Relationship between Selected Religious Norms and Drinking Behavior. Unpublished Ph.D. dissertation, Yale University, 1957.

Skolnick, Jerome H. Religious affiliation and drinking behavior. *Quarterly Journal of Studies on Alcohol*, 1958, *19*, 452-470.

Smith, Christopher J. and Hanham, Robert Q. *Alcohol Abuse: Geographical Perspectives*. Washington, DC: Association of American Geographers, 1982.

Smith, W. E. *The Word of Wisdom: A Test of the Predictability of Human Behavior*. Provo, UT: Brigham Young University, 1969.

Snyder, Charles R. *Alcohol and the Jews: A Cultural Study of Drinking and Sobriety*. Glencoe, IL: Free Press, 1958.

Snyder, Charles R. Culture and Jewish Sobriety: The Ingroup-Outgroup Factor. In: Pittman, David., and Snyder, Charles R. (eds.) *Society, Culture, and Drinking Patterns*. New York: John Wiley & Sons, 1962. pp. 188-229.

Snyder, Charles R. and Landman, R. H. Studies of drinking in Jewish culture. II. Prospectus for sociological research on Jewish drinking patterns. *Quarterly Journal of Studies on Alcohol*, 1951, *12*, 451-474.

Snyder, Charles R., Palgi, Phyllis, Eldar, Pnina, and Elian, Beatrice. Alcoholism among the Jews in Israel: A pilot study. I. Research rationale and a look at the ethnic factor. *Journal of Studies on Alcohol*, 1982, *43*, 623-654.

Spiegel, Marcia C. Profile of the alcoholic Jew. *British Journal of Alcohol and Alcoholism*, 1981, *16*, 141-149.

Spradley, James P. *You Owe Yourself a Drunk: An Ethnography of Urban Nomads*. Boston: Little, Brown, 1970.

Stevenson, Robert L. *The Works of Robert Louis Stevenson*. Vol. 18. *In the South Seas*. London: Chatto and Windus, 1912.

Stivers, Richard. *A Hair of the Dog: Irish Drinking and American Stereotype*. University Park, PA: Pennsylvania State University Press, 1976.

Stivers, Richard. Irish ethnicity and alcohol use. *Medical Anthropology*, 1978, *2*, 121-135.

Stivers, Richard. Historical Meanings of Irish-American Drinking. In: Bennett, Linda A., and Ames, Genevieve M. (eds.) *The American Experience with Alcohol: Contrasting Cultural Perspectives*. New York: Plenum, 1985. pp. 109-129.

Stout, David B. *San Blas Cuna Acculturation: An Introduction*. New York: Viking Fund Publications in Anthropology, 1947.

Straus, Robert, and Bacon, Selden D. *Drinking in College*. New Haven, CT: Yale University Press, 1953.

Sue, S., Kitano, H., Hatanaka, H., and Yeung, W. T. Alcohol Consumption among Chinese in the United States. In: Bennett, Linda, and Ames, G. (eds.) *The American Experience with Alcohol*. New York: Plenum, 1985. pp. 359-371.

Sue, S., Zane, N., and Ito, J. Reported alcohol drinking patterns among Asian and Caucasian Americans. *Journal of Cross-Cultural Psychology*, 1979, *10*, 41-56.

Taylor, William B. *Drinking, Homicide and Rebellion in Colonial Mexican Villages*.

Stanford, CA: Stanford University Press, 1979.

Thorner, Isidor. Ascetic protestantism and alcoholism. *Psychiatry*, 1953, *16*, 167-176.

Ulman, A. D. Ethnic differences in the first drinking experience. *Social Problems*, 1960, *8*, 45-56.

Unkovic, Charles M., Adler, Rudolf J., and Miller, Susan E. A Contemporary Study of Jewish Alcoholism - The Significant Other Point of View. In: Blaine, Allan (ed.) *Alcoholism and the Jewish Community.* New York: Federation of Jewish Philanthropies of New York, 1980. pp. 167-185.

Vaillant, George. Cultural Factors in the Etiology of Alcoholism: A Prospective Study. In: Babor, Thomas F. (ed.) *Alcohol and Culture: Comparative Perspectives from Europe and America.* New York: New York Academy of Sciences, 1986. (Annals of the New York Academy of Sciences, vol. 472)

Waddell, Jack O. "Drink, friend": Social Contexts of Convivial Drinking and Drunkenness among Papago Indians in an Urban Setting. In: Chafetz, Morris (ed.) *Proceedings of the First Annual Institute on Alcohol Abuse and Alcoholism.* Rockville, MD: National Institute on Alcohol Abuse and Alcoholism 1973. pp. 237-251.

Waddell, Jack O. For individual power and social credit: The use of alcohol among Tucson Papagos. *Human Organization*, 1975, *34*, 9-15.

Wafer, Lionel. *A New Voyage and Description of the Isthmus of America.* Oxford, England: The Hakluyt Society, 1934.

Washburne, Chandler. *Primitive Drinking: A Study of the Uses and Functions of Alcohol in Preliterate Societies.* New York: College and University Press, 1961.

Weber, Max. *Ancient Judaism.* Translated and edited by Gerth, Hans H. and Martindale, Don. New York: Free Press, 1952.

Westermeyer, J. Options regarding alcohol use among the Chippewa. *American Journal of Orthopsychiatry*, 1972, *42*, 398-403.

Westermeyer, Joseph. Use of Alcohol and Opium by the Meo of Laos. In: Marshall, Mac (ed.) *Beliefs, Behaviors, & Alcoholic Beverages: A Cross-Cultural Survey.* Ann Arbor, MI: University of Michigan Press, 1979. pp. 289-296. Originally published in *American Journal of Psychiatry*, 1971, 8, 1019-1023.

Wiener, Carolyn. *The Politics of Alcoholism.* New Brunswick, NJ: Transaction Books, 1981.

Wilkinson, Rupert. *The Prevention of Drinking Problems: Alcohol Control and Cultural Influences.* New York: Oxford University Press, 1970.

Williams, P. D. and Straus, Robert. Drinking patterns of Italians in New Haven, I. *Quarterly Journal of Studies on Alcohol*, 1950, *11*, 51-91.

Wilson, Ross. *Scotch: Its History and Romance.* Devon, Scotland: David & Charles, 1973.

Wolff, Peter H. Ethnic differences in alcohol sensitivity. *Science*, 1972, *125*, 449-451.

Yamamuro, Bufo. Notes on Drinking in Japan. In: Marshall, Mac (ed.) *Beliefs, Behaviors, & Alcoholic Beverages: A Cross-Cultural Survey.* Ann Arbor, MI: University of Michigan Press, 1979. pp. 270-277. Originally published in *Quarterly Journal of Studies on Alcohol*, 1954, *15*, 491-498.

Yawney, Carole. Drinking Patterns and Alcoholism in Trinidad. In: Marshall, Mac (ed.) *Beliefs, Behaviors, & Alcoholic Beverages: A Cross-Cultural Survey.* Ann Arbor, MI: University of Michigan Press, 1979. pp. 94-107. Originally published in Henry, Frances (ed.) *McGill Studies in Caribbean Anthropology*, Occasional Paper Series No. 5, 1969.

Yeh, E. K., and Hwu, H. G. Alcohol Abuse Dependence in a Chinese Metropolis: Findings from an Epidemiological Study in Taipei City. Paper presented at the Third Pacific Congress on Psychiatry, Seoul, Korea, May 14-19, 1984. Cited by Yu, Elena S. H., and Liu. William T. Alcohol Use and Abuse among Chinese Americans, *Alcohol Health and Research World*, 1986/1987, 14-17 and 60-61.

Yu, Elena S. H., and Liu, William T. Alcohol use and abuse among Chinese-Americans. *Alcohol Health and Research World*, 1986/1987, 14-17 and 60-61.

Yu, Elena S.H., Liu, William T., Xia, Zhengyi, and Zhang, Mingyuan. Alcohol Use, Abuse, and Alcoholism among Chinese Americans: A Review of the Epidemiologic Data. In: Spiegler, Danielle, Tate, Diane, Aitken, Sherrie, and Christian, Charles (eds.) *Alcohol Abuse among U. S. Ethnic Minorities*. Rockville, MD: National Institute on Alcohol Abuse, and Alcoholism, 1985. pp. 329-341.

Zimberg, Sheldon. Sociopsychiatric perspectives on Jewish alcohol abuse: Implications for the prevention of alcoholism. *American Journal of Drug and Alcohol Abuse*. 1977, *4*, 571-579.

Zimberg, Sheldon. A Socio-Psychiatric Perspective on Jewish Alcohol Abuse. In: Blaine, Allan (ed.) *Alcoholism and the Jewish Community*. New York: Federation of Jewish Philanthropies of New York, 1980. pp. 203-223.

Zylman, Richard. OVERemphasis on alcohol may be costing lives. *The Police Chief*, 1974, *41*, pp. 64-67.

3

American Experiences with Alcohol and Resulting Approaches to Reducing Alcohol Problems

In the early period of American life alcohol was widely and heavily consumed. Regular use was seen as healthful for everyone, including children, and alcohol problems were few. However, social and economic problems associated with the developing industrialization, urbanization, social conflict and social change increasingly became attributed to alcohol abuse and then to any use of beverage alcohol. A powerful prohibition movement ultimately succeeded in having a disastrous prohibition imposed on the nation. The prohibitionist tradition is found today in the control-of-consumption approach, which asserts that the more available alcohol is the more it will be consumed and that it is the quantity of alcohol consumed (rather than the manner of consumption, the norms surrounding consumption, behavioral expectations, etc.) that determines the extent of drinking problems. The approach is based on speculation which is unsupported by the body of available evidence. Even if control-of-consumption policies were to be effective in lowering mean per capita consumption, it is doubtful if drinking problems associated with heavy drinking would be reduced. Importantly, given the apparent health benefits and contribution to longevity of the moderate consumption of alcohol compared to abstinence, lowering the mean per capita consumption of alcohol among moderate drinkers could be highly undesirable for the health and longevity of this vast majority of the population. Thus, the control-of-consumption approach to alcohol problems should be rejected.

AMBIVALENCE TOWARD ALCOHOL

The place of alcohol in American society has long been ambivalent (Pittman, 1991, p. 776; Mecca, 1980, pp. 4-6; Christie, 1974, p. 9). "Drinking has been blessed and cursed, has been held the cause of economic catastrophe and the hope for prosperity, the major cause of crime, disease and military defeat, depravity and a sign of high prestige, mature personality, and a refined civilization" (Straus and Bacon, 1953). This ambivalence, which has been described as an extreme love-hate relationship (Milgram, 1990, p. 27), is not only societal, but often individual.

You have asked me how I feel about whiskey, a Mississippi state senator told his legislature in 1958. All right, here is just how I stand on this question:

If, when you say whiskey, you mean the devil's brew, the poison scourge, the bloody monster that defiles innocence, yea, literally takes the bread from the mouths of little children; if you mean the evil drink that topples the Christian man and woman from the pinnacles of righteous, gracious living into the bottomless pit of degradation and despair, shame and helplessness and hopelessness, then certainly I am against it with all of my power.

But if, when you say whiskey, you mean the oil of conversation, the philosophic wine, the stuff that is consumed when good fellows get together, that puts a song in their hearts and laughter on their lips and the warm glow of contentment in their eyes; if you mean Christmas cheer; if you mean the stimulating drink that puts the spring in the old gentleman's step on a frosty morning; if you mean the drink that enables a man to magnify his joy, and his happiness, and to forget, if only for a little while, life's great tragedies and heartbreaks and sorrows, if you mean that drink, the sale of which pours into our treasuries untold millions of dollars, which are used to provide tender care for our little children, our blind, our deaf, our dumb, our pitiful aged and infirm, to build highways, hospitals and schools, then certainly I am in favor of it.

This is my stand. I will not retreat from it; I will not compromise (Gross, 1983, pp. 23-24).

Organized efforts to limit drinking or the role of alcoholic beverages have existed in the United States since the early 1800s. However, alcohol has been the only substance whose proposed prohibition has provoked strong controversy and conflict. On one hand, the prohibition of narcotics has met little organized resistance, while the prohibition of cigarette, coffee or cola beverages sales has not attracted significant political support. Gusfield (1962, 1963) contends that alcohol has been a symbolic issue through which a struggle for primacy in social status has been fought between differing life styles--small town versus city, "old American" versus recent immigrant, the South and Midwest versus the Northeast. An alternate explanation is that while alcohol is clearly associated with numerous personal and social problems (thus motivating the prohibition impulse), its use is widespread and widely accepted (thus motivating its defense). In either case, the consequence is often intense emotion and social struggle.

At least as far back as the middle of the last century, the so-called temperance movement[1] widely began to preach the belief that all consumption of alcohol was evil and that the only solution for the problems resulting in alcohol misuse was the complete and total prohibition of the production, distribution, and consumption of alcohol. While the movement's success in imposing national Prohibition earlier in this century was a short-lived failure, its basic message continues to this day (Mecca, 1980, p. 5). Bacon and Jones (1968, p. 2) argue that "all thinking on the subject of alcohol in this country has been dominated for generations, and is still dominated to a large extent, by what came to be called the 'Wet-Dry controversy.'" While Prohibition was politically defeated, many of the beliefs, attitudes, and emotional reactions that supported it endure.

The chief legacy of this conflict has been a tendency to view all questions on the subject of alcohol in black-and-white terms of right and wrong, good and evil. Under the influence of the Wet-Dry controversy, the question of drinking became an either-or proposition. Either one drank, or one abstained. As a result, drinking and abstinence have come to be thought of as opposites on a scale of bad and good. Abstinence became associated in people's minds with purity and moral strength; drinking, with evil, disease, and degradation. All drinking has been assumed to hold the threat of loss of control and alcohol addiction. And, in the pattern of this thinking, the only effective means of dealing with the problems of alcohol has been to label all drinking as immoral and dangerous, and to pass laws against it (Bacon and Jones, 1968, p. 3).

After examining the American past, Zinberg and Fraser (1985, p. 460) concluded, "This culture, much more than others, has always behaved with great ambivalence toward the *idea* of alcohol use; . . . its historical record reveals numerous clearly identifiable and constantly changing rules and customs that deal with the reality of use" (emphasis in original). This ambivalence is reflected in the changing drinking age laws and drinking ethos indicated in Table 3.1.

ALCOHOL USE HAS CHANGED OVER TIME

During the first century and a half (1620-1775) of American life, alcohol was widely and heavily used. Toddlers drank beer, wine and cider with their parents, and regular use was seen as healthful for everyone (Asbury, 1950, pp. 3-4; Sinclair, 1962, pp. 36-37; Popham, 1978, pp. 267-277). For more than 30 years, because of this belief, abstainers had to pay one life insurance company rates 10% higher than that for drinkers. This was because the abstainer was considered "thin and watery, and as mentally cranked, in that he repudiated the good creatures of God as found in alcoholic drinks" (Kobler, 1973, p. 26).
    Alcohol was very important in this period:

Central to the drinking culture of colonial life was the tavern (used here as a term to cover inns, taverns, and ordinaries--any licensed establishment where alcohol was served on the premises). The role of the tavern in colonial America and the attitudes toward it were quite different from what they would become in the nineteenth century. The tavern was considered an integral part of community life, second only in importance to the meetinghouse, which served as the church, town hall, and courtroom. The laws of most

TABLE 3.1

A Schemata of Drinking Age Laws in the United States from 1700 to 1987 Relative to Drinking Ethos and Social Climate

Time	Age Law	Drinking Ethos	Social Climate
1700-1800	No age laws except in a few locale very young.	Colonial North America thrives on drinking. Men, women and children all use alcohol. Moderation is a cultural norm.	Rural life in the colonies. Close family ties. Parents had absolute authority to define children's rights and restrictions.
1800-1850	Isolated state and local laws began to evolve. The age varied, but usually was 16 or younger.	Drinking was beginning to change. Moderation was waning, and young (especially college youth) often drank heavily and sometimes engaged in delinquent behavior.	Industrial Revolution. Temperance Movement emerging.
1850-1920	Many local and state laws began to "protect youth" by age laws which varied from 16 to 20.	Temperance Movement flourishing and is not a major political force. Heavy drinking also continued.	16 to 20 year olds now being treated as preadolescents. Industrial development and job specialization put youth out of market.
1920-1930	Prohibition for all by constitutional amendment.	Drinking illegal, consumption moves underground. Mobster control of manufacture and distribution. Drinking continues in contempt of the law.	Nightlife flourishes in hidden bars and ballrooms. Unsettled period leading to economic depression.

Time	Age Law	Drinking Ethos	Social Climate
1934-1960	Age 21 established for postprohibition alcohol use.	Drinking continuing with alcohol now legal. Underage drinking now "a problem" as teenagers drink outside adult sanction.	Recovery from economic depression. World War II and baby boom of postwar period.
1960-1972	Many states lower drinking age to 18.	Alcohol use flourishes along with use of marijuana and other drugs.	Youth participation in economy and society very evident. Issues made over 18 as age of majority with all rights expected. Vietnam. "Hippie Movement."
1972-	States began moving drinking age back to 21. In 1986, Congress passes a law requiring all states to set 21 as legal age or lose highway funds.	Alcohol use flourishes with 75% of teenagers declaring that they use in national studies.	Negative reaction to high rate of youth involvement in drinking-related auto accidents. Republican administration and conservative movement in U.S. society.

Reprinted from the *International Journal of the Addictions* 23, pp. 631–632 by courtesy of Marcel Dekker Inc.

colonies required towns to license suitable persons to sell wine and spirits for the convenience of travelers and town dwellers; failure to do so could result in a fine. Contrary to the modern practice of keeping alcohol outlets a certain distance from schools and churches, colonial taverns were often required to be located near the meetinghouse or church. In towns that lacked a meetinghouse or in those where the meetinghouse did not provide sufficient warmth in winter, "religious services and court sessions were held in the great room of the principal tavern; there, ecclesiastical affairs were managed, the town selectmen and county justices met to conduct the business of government, and the voters assembled for town meetings" (Popham, 1978, p. 271). Those who attended these gatherings naturally took advantage of the hospitality of the tavern, the expenses not infrequently being paid out of town funds. People also came to taverns to see plays and concerts, to attend lodge meetings, to participate in lotteries, to read newspapers, and to engage in political debate. Taverns were, in fact, more important as centers of social activity than as places in which to drink. Most drinking took place in the home or at communal gatherings (Popham, 1978, pp. 267-277; Conroy, 1984) (Prendergast, 1987, p. 27).

The Revolutionary War saw the relaxation of antidrunkenness ordinances and an increase in alcohol problems. "Between 1790 and 1830 almost every aspect of American life underwent alteration, in many cases startling upheaval" (Rorabaugh, 1979, p. 125; also Levine, 1980, p. 32; Fallding, 1974, p. 26). Drinking, which had been controlled by the tightly knit family and social fabric in the colonial period, increasingly became an individualistic activity associated with masculine aggression and anti-social behavior by the early nineteenth century (Peele, 1987, p. 69). It became segregated by gender and age, which encouraged excessive consumption, and concern was frequently expressed over immoderate drinking. With the passage of time many of the problems associated with industrialization were perceived to be the result of alcohol abuse. "Middle- and upper-class Americans cut back their drinking drastically because it was no longer considered appropriate for an industrious life. As alcohol was eliminated from the ordinary daily routines of the middle class, when people did drink, they were more likely to go on binges where they drank all out" (Peele, 1989, p. 36).

With the settling of the West (which brought the moderating influence of women and children) drunkenness became less acceptable. "As social conditions improved there was a greater capacity for a reasonable family life, and alcohol was used less as a relief from intolerable conditions. At the same time, the level of emotionalism attached to drinking particularly the concept of machismo--male superiority shown in the capacity to hold liquor--began to drop" (Zinberg and Fraser, 1985, p. 467). The great waves of European immigration also had a moderating influence (Asbury, 1950, p. 1). Ironically, as moderate drinking patterns were re-established, prohibitionism grew in power and influence (Strayton, 1923, p. 34).

PROHIBITION MOVEMENT BECAME POWERFUL

The Women's Christian Temperance Union (WCTU), the National Temperance Society and Publication House, the Anti-Saloon League and other abstinence groups flooded the country with abstinence speakers, books, pamphlets, posters and curricular materials. And a flood it was; between 1865 and 1925, the Publication House alone printed over a billion pages of temperance literature (Kobler, 1973, p. 98). But that output was dwarfed by the Anti-Saloon League's American Issue Publishing House, established in 1909. Within three years of its creation, American Issue was producing about 250,000,000 book pages per month. And the quantity increased yearly. The WCTU and the Methodist Book Concern together appear to have produced as much material as American Issue, and there were innumerable smaller organizations that produced prohibitionist books, charts, leaflets, folders, pamphlets and sermons (Asbury, 1950, pp. 96-97).

In the decades following the Civil War, increasing veneration for science occurred and medical research on the effects of alcohol flourished. Temperance groups capitalized on this interest and activity by selectively publicizing research findings. But only those that supported the abstinence view were reported; those that supported moderate use were seen as biased, faulty or erroneous.

The drys perfected techniques for misrepresenting scientific experiments, for quoting out of context, for making final dogmas out of interim reports, and for manufacturing literary water bottles out of laboratory test tubes (Sinclair, 1962, pp. 38-39).

Temperance materials made no distinction between drinking and alcohol abuse, which were portrayed as one and the same. A typical poster presented the virtue and blessings of the abstainer on one side and the sin and misery of the drinker (synonymous with the drunk) on the other. The textbooks prepared by the WCTU reflected the view that "any quantity of alcohol in any form was toxic and when consumed regularly produced inheritable disorders into the third generation" (Kobler, 1973, p. 140). Suggested classroom demonstrations included putting part of a calf's brain in an empty jar into which alcohol would then be poured. The color of the brain would turn from pink to gray, and pupils would then be warned that a drink of alcohol would do the same to their brains (Kobler, 1973, p. 140).

The WCTU's Department of Scientific Temperance Instruction taught as scientifically proved fact that:

The majority of beer drinkers die from dropsy.

When it [alcohol] passes down the throat it burns off the skin leaving it bare and burning.

It causes the heart to beat many unnecessary times and after the first dose the heart is in danger of giving out so that it needs something to keep it up and, therefore, the person to whom the heart belongs has to take drink after drink to keep his heart going.

It turns the blood to water.

[Referring to invalids], A man who never drinks liquor will get well, where a drinking man would surely die (Kobler, 1973, p. 143).

The WCTU promoted compulsory temperance education so as to create "trained haters of alcohol[2] to pour a whole Niagara of ballots upon the saloon" (Sinclair, 1962, pp. 43-44). To this end it required that textbooks which it approved "teach that 'alcohol is a dangerous and seductive poison'; that fermentation turns beer and wine and cider from a food into poison; that a little liquor creates by its nature the appetite for more; and that degradation and crime result from alcohol" (Sinclair, 1962, p. 44). At least one-fourth of each book had to consist of temperance teaching, and publishers tended to have difficulty selling textbooks which were not approved by the WCTU. Many of the statements in approved texts were, at best, misleading and designed to frighten young impressionable readers:

A cat or dog may be killed by causing it to drink a small quantity of alcohol. A boy once drank whisky from a flask he had found, and died in a few hours. . . .

Alcohol sometimes causes the coats of the blood vessels to grow thin. They are then liable at any time to cause death by bursting. . . .

It often happens that the children of those who drink have weak minds or become crazy as they grow older. . . .

Worse than all, when alcohol is constantly used, it may slowly change the muscles of the heart into fat. Such a heart cannot be so strong as if it were all muscle. It is sometimes so soft that a finger could easily be pushed through its walls. You can think what would happen if it is made to work a little harder than usual. It is liable to stretch and stop beating and this would cause sudden death (Sinclair, 1962, p. 45).

Kobler (1973, p. 140) pointed out:

Nowhere in all this gallimaufry of misguidance . . . aimed at children, or in any of the prohibition literature and talk addressed to adults, did there linger the ghost of a suggestion that perhaps one might drink moderately without damage to oneself or to others. The very word "moderation" inflamed the WCTU and the Prohibition Party. It was "the shoddy life-belt, which promises safety, but only tempts into danger, and fails in the hour of need . . . the fruitful fountain from which the flood of intemperance is fed. . . . Most men become drunkards by trying to drink moderately and failing." Even conceding that a rare few could conceivably imbibe in moderation at no risk to themselves, they should nevertheless refrain lest they set a bad example for the weaker majority of the human race.

Little wonder that even today Americans tend to treat alcohol with the same caution as guns, drugs and germs (Honigman, 1979, p. 415) and that many tend to feel guilty when they have even a single drink (Sinclair, 1962, p. 46).

In each American temperance cycle of the past, reformers typically tried to reform drinkers by persuasion, but finally resorted to legal coercion (Blocker,

1989).

A confluence of many factors, in addition to the avalanche of propaganda, made possible such coercion through the passage of the Eighteenth Amendment establishing national Prohibition. These included the effective lobbying of well-organized temperance organizations, the argument that the alcohol beverage industry diverted foodstuffs needed for the war effort, the association of alcohol with "threatening" new urban immigrants, the lack of organization on the part of "wets," and political intimidation (Kobler, 1973, ch. 9; Asbury, 1950, ch. 7; Kerr, 1985, ch. 6). Few of the wets could conceive of a dry America; they lost by default (Kobler, 1973, p. 205).

The "great experiment" of Prohibition (1920-1933) is generally recognized as a failure. Not only did it fail to prevent the consumption of alcohol, but it led to the extensive production of unregulated and untaxed alcohol, the development of organized crime empires, increased violence, massive political corruption and widespread contempt for law (Engelmann, 1979; Kobler, 1973, ch. 10-13; Sinclair, 1962, ch. 9-15; Asbury, 1950, ch. 9-14; Everest, 1978; Grant and Ritson, 1983, p. 21; Nelli, 1985). Thus, it was ineffective and counter-productive, just as it proved to be in Iceland (1919-1932), Russia (1916-1917), Finland (1919-1932) (Ewing and Rouse, 1976), and elsewhere around the world (Marshall, 1979, p. 456; Heath, 1987, p. 46).[3]

Nevertheless, as Zimmer and Morgan (1992) point out, some writers have more recently argued that Prohibition had positive health consequences. Such writers (Aaron and Musto, 1981; Burnham, 1968; Gerstein, 1981; Kyvig, 1985; Moore, 1989) generally rely on data compiled by Warburton (1932) and Emerson (1932). However, Warburton's data "clearly show that cirrhosis deaths began to decline as early as 1907, well before federal prohibition, and actually increased slightly during the latter years of prohibition," explain Zimmer and Morgan (1992, p. 1), who add "Emerson's cirrhosis data show a decline beginning in 1911, a more dramatic decline in the preprohibition years (1916-1919), and a slight increase during prohibition. Following prohibition's repeal, cirrhosis death rates were relatively stable until 1942 when they began to rise" (also see Miron and Zweibel, 1991). Furthermore, "The increase in the cirrhosis rate from 1922-1933 was also accompanied by similar increases in alcoholism deaths and alcohol psychosis" (Zimmer and Morgan, 1992, p. 1). They (p. 2) continue "We do not know if the increase in these adverse consequences was related to an increase in the number of drinkers or increased consumption of alcohol by a portion of those who drank illegally. What we do know is that consumption of distilled spirits increased during prohibition reversing a century long trend toward beer and wine" (Hyman et al., 1980; Rorabaugh, 1979; Levine, 1984).

This shift in marketing and consumption to more potent forms of intoxicant has been called the iron law of prohibition (Cowan, 1986). Distilled spirits are more easily smuggled and concealed than beer or wine.

PROHIBITION WAS COUNTER-PRODUCTIVE

Prohibition encouraged the rapid consumption of high-proof drinks in secretive, non-socially regulated and controlled ways. "People did not take the trouble to go to a speakeasy, present the password, and pay high prices for very poor quality alcohol simply to have a beer. When people went to speakeasies, they went to get drunk" (Zinberg and Fraser, 1985, p. 468). Zinberg and Fraser (1985, p. 470) conclude: "Removing alcohol from the norms of everyday society increased drinking problems. Without well-known prescriptions for use and commonly held sanctions against abuse, Prohibition drinkers were left almost as defenseless as were the South American Indians in the face of Spanish rum and brandy." They (1985, p. 470) suggest that Prohibition "may have curtailed the growth of the responsible drinking practices that had emerged during the 25 or so years preceding passage of the Volstead Act."[4]

The repeal of Prohibition returned control over alcohol to the states, where it largely remained until the establishment of the National Institute on Alcohol Abuse and Alcoholism (NIAAA) in 1972. Under the leadership of Dr. Morris Chafetz, the NIAAA promoted a policy of encouraging responsible drinking for those who chose to drink (Chafetz, 1974, p. xiii). Thus, it adhered to a socio-cultural approach to reducing alcohol abuse.

ALTERNATIVE APPROACHES TO REDUCING ALCOHOL PROBLEMS

Philosophies and approaches to reducing drinking problems can be generally categorized as being socio-culturally oriented or control-of-consumption oriented. The socio-cultural model tends to assume that

1) It is the misuse of alcohol, not alcohol itself, that is the source of drinking problems.
2) It is important to distinguish between drinking and alcohol abuse.[5]
3) The misuse of alcohol can be reduced by educating individuals to make one of two decisions:
   - one decision is to abstain;
   - the other decision is to drink responsibly.
4) Because many individuals will choose to drink alcohol, it is important that societal norms regarding what is acceptable and unacceptable behavior for those who choose to drink be clear and unambiguous.
5) People who are going to drink as adults should gradually learn how to drink.[6]

The socio-cultural approach is reflected in the following proposals:

1) Raise minimum drinking age laws and include provisions permitting parents

to serve their children alcohol so that young people who choose to drink can learn to do so in a moderate, controlled manner and in a safe, caring environment.

2) Provide objective alcohol education that presents moderation in drinking, rather than drinking itself, as an indicator of maturity.

3) Modify governmental regulations to encourage advertising that portrays alcohol not as a magical potion but as an enjoyable part of ordinary life and to be consumed in moderation.

4) Change tax laws to encourage consumption of lighter-proof beverages consumed with food.

5) Eliminate the stigmatization of alcohol.

6) Modify licensing laws and alcohol regulations so as to encourage consumption in family-oriented, rather than drinking-only, settings (Wilkinson, 1970).

On the other hand, the control-of-consumption model tends to assume that

1) The substance of alcohol is the necessary and sufficient cause of all drinking problems.

2) The availability of alcohol determines the extent to which it will be consumed.

3) The quantity of alcohol consumed (rather than the manner in which it is consumed, the purpose for which it is consumed, the social context in which it is consumed, etc.) determines the extent of drinking problems.

4) Educational efforts should be directed toward stressing the problems that alcohol consumption can cause and encouraging abstinence.

The more traditional control-of-consumption approach called for the complete and total prohibition of the manufacture, distribution, sale, possession and consumption of any and all alcoholic beverages. Given the demonstrated failure of prohibition,[7] adherents of the control-of-consumption model now more typically call for a diversity of measures designed to discourage consumption. These include such policies as imposing higher taxes on alcoholic beverages, limiting or reducing the number of sales outlets, further restricting the permissible location for sales outlets, limiting the alcoholic content of beverages, prohibiting or limiting the advertising of alcohol, requiring the use of warning messages with all advertisements and on all beverage containers, requiring the display of warning signs in establishments that sell or serve alcoholic beverages, limiting the days or hours during which alcohol can be sold, increasing server liability for subsequent problems associated with the misuse of alcohol, limiting the sale of alcohol to people of specific ages, decreasing the legal alcohol blood content level for driving vehicles and eliminating the tax deductibility of alcohol as a business expense.

The control-of-consumption approach assumes that the problem is alcohol,[8] while the sociocultural approach assumes that the misuse of alcohol is the problem. Hence, the control-of-consumption policies attempt to prevent or discourage people from consuming alcohol, while socio-cultural policies attempt to prevent people from using alcohol irresponsibility.

The control-of-consumption approach is "based not on an understanding of the reasons why people begin to drink, why most who drink do not have alcohol problems, and why some individuals or subgroups develop pathological drinking patterns, but on the belief that if alcoholic beverages are made less available and attractive through governmental intervention, then fewer people will become alcohol abusers or alcoholics" (Pittman, 1980, p. 3). It is a prohibitionistic orientation "based on the simplistic stance that alcohol causes alcohol problems, and to eliminate the latter we must first eliminate beverage alcohol's easy availability" (Pittman, 1980, p. 4; also see Herd, 1992, p. 1121).

ALCOHOL STIGMATIZED BY CONTROL-OF-CONSUMPTION ADVOCATES

As indicated above, the NIAAA originally promoted the socio-cultural approach. However, by the late 1970s, under the direction of Ernest Nobel, it adopted the control-of-consumption approach (National Institute on Alcohol Abuse and Alcoholism, 1978). In Nobel's opinion, "Alcohol is the dirtiest drug we have. It permeates and damages all tissue. No other drug can cause the same degree of harm that it does. Not even marijuana, heroin or LSD, as dirty and dangerous as they are, are as pervasive in the damage they cause as alcohol" (Ford, 1988, p. 176). The Institute's deputy director has publicly asserted that there is no such thing as responsible drinking, and the secretary of the Department of Health and Human Services has directed all agencies under his direction to replace the phrase "substance abuse" with "alcohol and other drug abuse" (Ford, 1988, p. 176). The federal Office for Substance Abuse Prevention's editorial guidelines (New York State Division of Alcoholism and Alcohol Abuse, n.d., p. 77) include the following:

Do Not Use	Use
Substance abuse	Alcohol and other drug abuse
Substance use	Alcohol and other drug use
Abuse when sentence refers to youth, teens, or children (anyone under 21)	Use (DHHS aims to prevent the the use, not abuse, of alcohol and other drugs by youth)
Responsible use	Use (since there is risk associated with all use)
Drunk driving (because a person does not have to be drunk to be impaired)	Alcohol-impaired driving

Do Not Use	Use
Accidents when referring	Crashes (since the term
to alcohol and other	"accident" suggests the
drug use	event could not have
	been avoided)

Although abstinence is the goal of the "Just Say No" approach, other "Language of Prevention" guidelines warn, "Use of the term 'abstinence' frequently evokes a negative response. Whenever possible the Division [of Alcoholism and Alcohol Abuse] suggests alternatives such as 'non-use' or 'choosing not to use' as more positive . . ." (New York State Division of Alcoholism and Alcohol Abuse, n.d.a, p. 9).

These guidelines reflect OSAP's position "that for kids under 21, there is no difference between alcohol or other drug *use* and *abuse*" (Office for Substance Abuse Prevention, 1989, p. 10, emphases in original).[9]

In its *Drug Prevention Education: A Guide to Selection and Implementation*, the U.S. Department of Education (1988, pp. 10-11) asserts that curricular materials should present "a clear and consistent message that the use of alcohol, tobacco, and other illicit drugs is unhealthy (sic) and harmful"[10] and warns that in some curricula that message "is lost altogether as publishers strive to balance conflicting views. . . ." Educators selecting a curriculum are also specifically warned:

Curricula which advocate *"responsible use"* of drugs should be rejected. Such curricula tend to foster a belief that some illicit drugs, especially marijuana, are not particularly harmful if used in moderation. Yet we know from research that marijuana and other drugs, including alcohol and tobacco, can have devastating effects, especially on developing bodies. While today's curricula seldom urge "responsible use" in the same explicit fashion as those marketed in the 1970s, consumers should be alert to curricula which rely even implicitly on camouflaged versions of this theory.

For example, pay attention if a curriculum tells students that drugs themselves are neither good nor bad, but that *how* they are used is the most important factor.

Another warning sign is the "some believe this . . . while others believe that" approach which avoids being "judgmental" about drugs. Phrases like "research is inconclusive" or "not enough is known to make a judgment" about the effects of drugs are red flags. There is a wealth of conclusive research about the harmful effects of drugs, and curricula should not waffle on this point. Any curriculum which contains unclear messages about using dangerous substances should be rejected (U. S. Department of Education, 1988, pp. 10-11, ellipses and emphasis in original).[11]

Alcohol: the Gateway Drug, New York State's curriculum guide for kindergarten through grade 12, is consistent with federal policy:

Associated with the continued public acceptance of alcohol as a benign substance rather than a mind-altering, addictive drug is the concept of "responsible drinking. . . ."

While responsible drinking programs recognize that youth under the legal possession age are faced with choices about alcohol use, the strategy automatically presumes that the "normal" choice will be use. The message that non-use is the choice strongly preferred by society for young people is often overlooked, as is the fact that laws must be broken for young people to use alcohol except under parental supervision. The strategy also implies that responsible use is a way to prevent alcohol problems. The word "responsible" itself suggests that some "irresponsibility" is at the root of alcohol problems, something we *know* is inaccurate. Non-use is the only sure way to prevent alcohol problems (New York State Division of Alcoholism and Alcohol Abuse, n.d., p. 2 emphasis in original).

In referring to alcohol as a drug, control-of-consumption proponents are technically correct. Pharmacologically, "any substance that by its chemical nature alters structure or function in the living organism is a drug. . . . Pharmacological effects are exerted by foods, vitamins, hormones, microbial, metabolites, plants, snake venoms, stings, products of decay, air pollutants, pesticides, minerals, synthetic chemicals, virtually all foreign materials (very few are completely inert), and many materials normally in the body" (Modell, 1967, p. 345). However, their intent appears to be to stigmatize alcohol by associating it with illicit drugs. This is frequently accomplished by discussing alcohol in the same paragraph with crack cocaine and other illicit drugs. Often the effort is more direct. The Maine Department of Education (n.d.) states, "The term 'alcohol/drug' is used to emphasize that alcohol is a mind-altering drug needing equal consideration with all other mind-altering drugs," the Florida Department of Education refers to alcohol as a harmful drug (Morton, 1990, p. 6), Oregon's Department (Mielke and Holstedt, 1991, p. 472) states unequivocally that wine coolers are illegal drugs, and Georgia's Department (Georgia Department of Education, n.d., p. 15) contends, without any qualification, that alcohol is harmful to the body. A poster distributed by the New York State Division of Alcoholism and Alcohol Abuse (n.d.c) poses in large upper-case letters the question "DO YOU USE DRUGS?" above a picture of a bottle of beer; at the bottom it asserts: "More people get into trouble with alcohol than any other drug. Beer contains alcohol." Another poster warns in large letters above a bottle of wine cooler "Don't be fooled"; below it warns in large letters "This is a drug" (New York State Division of Alcoholism and Alcohol Abuse (n.d.d). The effort to stigmatize alcohol is even used effectively by some politicians. Consequently, producers are increasingly finding it necessary to explain how alcoholic beverages differ from illicit drugs (Rose, 1991, p. 104).

In stigmatizing alcohol, control proponents may inadvertently trivialize the use of illegal drugs and thereby encourage their use. Or, especially among younger students, they may create the false impression that parents who use alcohol in moderation are drug abusers whose good example they should reject. Thus, their misguided effort to equate alcohol with illicit drugs is likely to be counterproductive.

The U.S. Department of Education's rejection of the obvious fact that drugs themselves are neither good nor bad is unfortunate. Curricula that present some substances as inherently beneficial or detrimental in and of themselves are patently incorrect (Washburne, 1961, pp. 266-267) and will loose credibility, at least among more intelligent students.

An OSAP publication (Office for Substance Abuse Prevention, 1987, p. 11) describes alcohol as a poison and implies that drinking might lead to death.[12] Similarly, the State Education Department of New York (n.d., p. 30) defines alcohol as toxic. Another OSAP publication (1988, p. 16) asserts that the effects of alcohol (no level or degree of usage indicated) are that "[b]rain cells are altered and may die. Memory formation is blocked. . . . In men hormone levels change, causing lower sex drive and enlarged breasts. Women's menstrual cycles become irregular, and their ovaries malfunction. Deterioration of the heart muscle can occur."[13]

The same publication (p.17) presents "Four Basic Stages of Alcohol and Other Drug Use," according to which, in stage four, "Blackouts and overdosing are more common, family life is a disaster, and crime may be becoming a way of life. . . ." The presentation clearly implies a natural, if not inexorable, progression through the stages to a life of disaster.

Federal and state publications frequently describe alcohol as a "gateway drug" that will lead people into illicit drug use. The "evidence" is that most people who are involved with illicit drugs drank alcohol first. Of course, most illicit drug users also earlier drank milk, ate candy bars, and drank cola. Kaufman (1988, pp. 137-138) has pointed out:

The steppingstone hypothesis was controversially presented as a primary danger of marijuana in that it led to the use of "hard" drugs, particularly heroin. A major refutation of this theory has been that alcohol is a more common precursor and therefore a steppingstone to heroin dependence. Schut et al. showed that 97 of 100 heroin addicts reported using alcohol prior to illicit drugs. . . . We propose that neither alcohol nor marijuana are truly steppingstones in that they seduce a nonpredisposed individual down the path to "hard" drugs. Rather, they are both very commonly used in our society and are used and abused more frequently by those who eventually go on to "harder" drugs. However, the gateway hypothesis is presented as dramatic fact when it is an untested hypothesis which is extremely difficult to support or refute.

CONTROL-OF-CONSUMPTION MODEL IS NEO-PROHIBITIONIST

The control-of-consumption model is also known as the control, the control of production, the availability, the new temperance, the neo-Prohibitionist, the neo-dry, the public health and the single distribution model.

The relevance of all but the last two terms are obvious from the central assumptions of the approach: ". . . the greater the availability of alcohol in a society, the greater the prevalence and severity of alcohol-related problems in that society" (Single, 1988, p. 355). More specifically it assumes that

1) Alcohol availability is positively related to mean levels of consumption . . .
2) Mean consumption is related to levels of heavy drinking. . . .
3) Heavy drinking is associated with adverse health and social consequences . . . (Single, 1988, p. 326).

It has been pointed out that "[t]he availability of or easy access to alcoholic beverages at a low price are viewed as overriding forces that will in fact mitigate against human beings making responsible decisions about alcohol (Lauderdale, 1977, p. 3).

CONTROL-OF-CONSUMPTION ALSO CALLED PUBLIC HEALTH MODEL

The term "public health model" is sometimes used because the approach often rests upon the epidemiological model developed in public health for describing the transmission of illness within a population. For example, the concepts of agent, host and vector are useful in understanding the spread of malaria among humans. The infection is caused by the malarial protozoan (the agent), that typically enters the body of a human (the host) through bites from the anopheles mosquito (the vector). Malaria can be controlled by killing the agent (very difficult and impractical), immunizing the host, or destroying the vector (by destroying breeding swamps and engaging in large scale spraying) (Lauderdale, 1977, pp. 4-5).

It is clear that drinking alcohol is a necessary condition for either alcoholism or alcohol problems, and that totally eliminating alcohol would eliminate alcohol problems. However, the vast majority of people use alcohol without any difficulty and it is questionable that simply reducing availability would have any positive consequence. Alcohol doesn't "infect" people as microbes do; importantly, at moderate levels of consumption it appears to be beneficial to health and longevity. Thus, the epidemiological model appears to be highly inappropriate.

CONTROL-OF-CONSUMPTION OFTEN CALLED SINGLE DISTRIBUTION MODEL

The term "single distribution model" is also frequently used. The log normal distribution model, more commonly called the single distribution model, was proposed during the mid-1950s by a demographer, Sully Ledermann (1956).[14] Unlike the normal curve, the log normal curve cannot have negative values (people cannot drink less than nothing). It is skewed to the left, reflecting the fact that most drinkers consume at a moderate level, while proportionately fewer drinkers consume at progressively higher levels.

The Ledermann curve can be presented in graphic form with the abscissa being the amount of alcohol consumed in the population, and with the ordinate being either the number or percentage of drinkers. It is continuous and unimodel. See Figure 3.1.

It is assumed that the shape of the curve is invariant, i.e., attitudes, beliefs, cultural practices, beverage preferences, and other social variables have essentially no influence on the distribution or proportion of heavy drinkers, Importantly, "Ledermann's formulation is conspicuously atheoretical, i.e., there is no known logical reason for the shape of the curve or the relationship between mean consumption and the proportion of heavy drinkers" (Colón, 1979, pp. 11-12).

It is also assumed that knowledge of the mean consumption permits prediction of the proportion of heavy drinkers. Specifically, it is believed that if mean consumption is increased, the curve will move to the right and the number of persons at the right-hand end of the distribution will be increased. That is, there will be an increase in the number of heavy drinkers (Parker and Harman, 1978, p. 381). Importantly, one of the properties of the lognormal curve is that the proportion of heavy drinkers increases multiplicatively as the mean consumption level rises. Thus, for example, if mean consumption doubles, the number of heavy drinkers would increase roughly eightfold (Smith, 1985, p. 103).

FIGURE 3.1

The Ledermann Curve

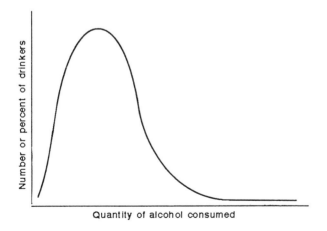

Note - Adapted from de Lint (1973. p.16).

Pittman has pointed out that

a major fallacy in the Ledermann assumption that alcohol consumption in a population has a constant pattern of distribution from those who abstain to those who are heavy imbibers of beverage alcohol. This assumption means that the researcher must accept as an article of faith that the distribution of alcohol consumption does not either change over time for a population or with the group being studied. This assumption is contradicted by longitudinal survey data of the drinking behavior of college students originally studied by Straus and Bacon in 1949-1951, being currently resurveyed by Bacon and associates approximately 25 years later, which finds dramatic changes in individual drinking patterns.

Thus it is essential to know the dispersion of consumption or the variance from the mean consumption, as drinking patterns and amounts consumed do vary by age, sex, race, religion, ethnicity, and other socio-cultural variables within a national population as well as between national populations.

. . . a major criticism of the Ledermann model is that its reliance on mean consumption as the only parameter needed to be known tells us nothing about the dispersion of consumption. It is quite possible for two populations to have the same mean consumption but to have radically different (high and low) dispersions in their distributions. Inferences derived from drinking surveys of subpopulations would dictate the assumption that the amount of absolute alcohol consumed by a total population can be distributed among consumers in quite different amounts (Pittman, 1980, p. 44).

An empirical problem is the fact that there are rarely enough data to test the goodness of fit among heavy drinkers (i.e., those on the far right side tail of the distribution). Importantly, those data that are available tend not to support the theory (Skog, 1973, p. 10; Duffy and Cohen, 1978; Parker and Harman, 1978).

The statistician Duffy succinctly points out a simple but major problem:

The Ledermann proposition, however formulated, is false, not only on account of shortcomings in parameter estimation and data sets adduced in support, etc., but because it is founded on the erroneous belief that a characteristic (in this case alcohol consumption) must follow a simple mathematical distribution. It has been demonstrated time and again in other fields that this is not so. . . . I do not doubt that the distribution of alcohol consumption is positively skewed in many cases, but it is neither smooth nor continuous, and there is not convincing evidence that it is unimodel (Duffy, 1978, pp. 1649-1650).

Another very serious problem is that "[c]urrent measures of beverage alcohol consumption are so beset with unresolved methodological and statistical problems in the areas of production, sales, and per capita consumption statistics that they should not be used to set the social policy goals of any society in reference to preventive programs for alcoholism and alcohol-related problems" (Pittman, 1980, p. 37).

CONTROL-OF-CONSUMPTION MODEL IS INADEQUATE

In spite of both logical (Alanko, 1992, pp. 3-5) and empirical evidence (Hilton and Clark, 1987, pp. 521-522) to the contrary, control theorists still insist that a decrease in the mean per capita consumption of alcohol will invariably lead to a decrease in heavy drinkers. It should now be obvious that this assumption is highly speculative and not based on scientific data (Pittman, 1980, p. 45).[15]

Even if their central assumption were true, control-of-consumption advocates focus exclusively on level of consumption and ignore other important variables. They incorrectly (Sadava, 1985, pp. 395-396; Gusfield, 1974, p. 98) assume that heavy drinking is directly and closely associated with alcoholism and health problems. However, even cirrhosis does not always show regular correlations with level of consumption. Heath (1982) compared the relatively heavy-drinking Navajo Indians, who evince little cirrhosis, with the neighboring Hopi, who consume less alcohol but have a far higher incidence of the malady. The more sober Hopi expel the few heavy-drinking members of their society into a rural Skid Row whose denizens drink themselves to death. Drinking has risen dramatically in Holland without a concomitant rise in liver cirrhosis (de Lint, 1981), whereas in Britain--which consumes somewhat more alcohol per capita than does the United States--the cirrhosis rate is about one-fifth of that in the United States (Sulkunen, 1976). "Differences in drinking problems for contiguous groups that are unrelated to the consumption levels of the groups are common. Bruun (1959), an advocate of alcohol controls, noted that there was no connection between quantity of alcohol consumed and the appearance of drinking problems in the small groups he observed in Finland" (Peele, 1987, p. 68). Peele also points out that compilation of countries according to their consumption of absolute alcohol at times almost exactly reverse the listings of countries according to their alcohol-related problems. Thus, the "wettest" countries tend to have less problem drinking and alcoholism while the "driest" tend to have the highest drinking problem rates (Peele, 1987, p. 67). Colón et al. (1981, pp. 357-358) report: "The posited exclusive relationship between alcoholism and consumption, the cornerstone of the single distribution model, was found to be accounted for by other variables in the present multivariate model. The lack of congruence among predictors of alcoholism and predictors of consumption is intrinsic to this finding. It should not be overlooked that the present study employed a definition of alcoholism based on physical pathology, cirrhosis, that, if anything, is favorable to the single distribution model." They conclude that "it is an oversimplification to view alcoholism merely as an extension of heavy drinking" (Colón et al., 1981, pp. 347-348). Even control advocate Mäkelä (1978, p. 344) has concluded that ". . . the available evidence indicates that there exist important cultural variations in the incidence of social consequences of drinking that are unrelated to the average level of consumption."

Control-of-consumption advocates almost universally ignore such obviously important factors as body weight, diet, and drinking patterns (e.g., steady or episodic) (Parker and Harman, 1979, p. 78). Thus, their simplistic model cannot adequately reflect the reality of a complex world.

CONTROL-OF-CONSUMPTION POLICIES MAY BE COUNTER-PRODUCTIVE

Importantly, "A question we hasten to raise is whether reducing per capita consumption through price control might not result in a change in drinking patterns from steady to episodic consumption, from greater frequency and total consumption to greater quantity consumed per occasion. We are seeking specifically if a set of policies that might reduce a chronic problem such as cirrhosis might not increase an acute problem such as cognitive impairment. Put another way, what are the unanticipated consequences of the control policy recommended by distribution theorists?" (Parker and Harman, 1979, p. 78). Similarly, Colón and Cutter (1983, p. 87) point out, "Curtailment of on-premise availability, for example, may bring about a modest curtailment in the liver cirrhosis death rate (Colón, 1981). Nevertheless, such curtailment simultaneously may have a far greater negative impact on mortality by increasing highway fatalities."

CONTROL-OF-CONSUMPTION POLICIES AND PROHIBITIONISM: HOW DIFFERENT?

It should be noted that the beliefs as well as the policies commonly promoted by control-of-consumption advocates appear to be virtually identical to those of the Anti-Saloon League and the American Temperance League (now combined and known as the American Council on Alcohol Problems) and similar groups. Consequently, it is difficult to differentiate between materials produced by such groups as the NIAAA and the American Council on Alcohol Problems or the National Temperance and Prohibition Council. For example, the American Council on Alcohol Problems asserts that "problems relating to alcohol and other drugs are in direct proportion to consumption. More consumers and higher per capita consumption produce increased problems . . ." and it advocates "activities aimed at reducing both the number of consumers of alcohol (and other drugs), and the per capita rate of consumption" (American Council on Alcohol Problems, n.d., p. 2). It takes pride in its role in

* Restoring "Age 21" laws for purchasing alcohol in all fifty states
* Mandating of warning labels on alcoholic beverage containers
* Increasing federal excise taxes on alcoholic beverages (American Council on Alcohol Problems, n.d., p. 2).

This abstinence group also strongly promotes other control measures, such as strict controls on alcohol advertising and marketing practices, including a ban on TV ads and mandated warning labels on all ads and promotions (American Council on Alcohol Problems, n.d., p. 2). The National Temperance and Prohibition Council similarly echoes the NIAAA in referring to alcohol as "a drug and a poison" (National Temperance and Prohibition Council, 1991, p. 1) and in its efforts "To emphasize the deceptiveness of the word 'abuse' [by] indicating the danger as being in alcohol and other drug *use*, not only its abuse" (National Temperance and Prohibition Council, n.d., p. 2, emphasis in original).

CONTROL-OF-CONSUMPTION POLICIES MAY BE DANGEROUS

Much research has been conducted to determine if various proposals advocated by control theorists (restricted outlets, higher alcohol prices, increased drinking ages, etc.) lead to lower consumption. However, given the speculative nature of the Ledermann distribution curve and its doubtful ability to predict the proportion of heavy drinkers, merely demonstrating a decrease in mean per capita consumption would appear to be irrelevant to the incidence of heavy drinking. Furthermore, *given the apparent health benefits and contribution to longevity of the moderate consumption of alcohol compared to either abstinence or heavy drinking, reducing per capita consumption might well have serious adverse health effects for moderate drinkers. Thus, lowering the mean per capita consumption of alcohol could be counterproductive and highly undesirable for the health and longevity of the general population.*

This problem can be seen in the issue of warning labels, which implicitly warn against any and all consumption of alcohol. Warning labels may be consistent with the agenda of new temperance workers, who seek to reduce per capita consumption across the board, but might not be consistent with the health and longevity of moderate drinkers. For this reason Ford (1988, p. 49) has suggested that warning labels conclude with the following statement: "Recognizing, however, that moderate use of this product may help to prevent cardiovascular and other life threatening diseases and add to the general well-being of the user." Interestingly, the Director of the NIAAA recently asserted: "Requiring health warning labels on alcoholic beverage containers is a good example of a policy enacted in an area where (sic) the scientific evidence is limited" (Gordis, 1991, p. 102). However, it would appear to date that warning labels have no impact discernable on either moderate or problem drinkers (Graves, 1992, pp. 14-15).

CONTROL-OF-CONSUMPTION POLICIES QUESTIONABLE

Rush et al. (1986) and Gliksman and Rush (1986) found evidence suggesting some relationship between availability and consumption as well as between sociodemographic variables and consumption. However, both studies suffer serious methodological weaknesses (Moskowitz, 1989, p. 58). Holder and Blose (1987) found stronger evidence of a relationship between permitting alcohol-by-the-drink for on-premises consumption and increased drinking. Frankel and Whitehead (1985) conclude that the evidence concerning the relationship between overall consumption of alcohol and the number of alcohol outlets is inconclusive. They suggest that the hours during which alcohol could be sold affects drinking patterns (i.e., when and where it is consumed), but not the rate or total amount of alcohol consumed.

State or provincial restrictions on the availability of alcohol do not appear to reduce alcohol-related problems. Reviews of the literature (for example Smart, 1977; Popham et al., 1978; Harford et al., 1979; Rabow and Watts, 1982) suggest that the relationship is nonexistent, small, or equivocal.

Simon (1966, p. 193) concluded that ". . . the number of outlets is more likely to respond to consumption, rather than to be the cause of consumption," and Entine (1963) found that outlets tended to follow population movements, a fact which tends to support Simon's conclusion.

Bacon (1971) found little relationship between a collective measure of availability and alcohol consumption, and Smart (1976, 1977) found none. Fillmore and Whitman (1982, p. 12) found that despite an increase in the availability of alcohol, college students reported remarkable stability in their drinking patterns. Similarly, Drew (1979) found that while the per capita consumption of alcohol increased about 15% in Australia between 1952 and 1977, this *increase* was accompanied by an equivalent *decrease* in highway fatalities.

In 1985, Iowa abandoned its state monopoly on beverage alcohol and the resulting shift to a private distribution system "constituted the most abrupt and dramatic increase in alcohol availability that any state has experienced since the repeal of Prohibition" (Mulford et al., 1992, p. 487). The number of outlets exploded and alcohol quickly became available in nearly all grocery and convenience stores. Additionally, "Sunday sales were legalized, hours of sales were extended, advertising was allowed and purchases could be made on credit terms" (Mulford et al., 1992, p. 487).

To assess the impact of this dramatic increase in availability, Mulford and Fitzgerald (1988) compared both wine sales and self-reported wine consumption both before and after the change. They found that after an increase immediately following the de-control, monthly wine sales steadily declined to control levels. Self-reported wine consumption nine months after the change were the same as that identified four months before the change. A second study (Mulford et al., 1992) included data on spirits. The researchers reported: "Time series analyses of monthly sales (apparent consumption) trends showed that the increased availability had no lasting impact on consumption" (Mulford et al., 1992, p. 487).

Unfortunately, not all research is so apparently benign. For example, a study of every town or city with a population of at least 10,000 in the state of Tennessee explored the relationship between the availability of alcohol (indicated by ordinances governing sale of alcohol and number of alcohol outlets per 100,000 population) and several deleterious behaviors and conditions. The investigators (Dull and Giacopassi, 1986, pp. 518-519) found that the tougher the control, the greater the abuse and reported that their

. . . data give support to the "forbidden fruit" hypothesis whereby stricter ordinances actually lead to an increase in socially undesirable alcohol-related phenomena. On the basis of our data, it appears doubtful that tighter restrictions on alcohol availability will alleviate these problems. We would concur with Room's (1971) conclusion that government policies are not necessarily producing their intended effects. If anything, the relation seems to be that the more restrictive the policy, the higher the rate of drinking related problems. It is quite conceivable that, if the "forbidden fruit" hypothesis is correct, such legislative efforts to limit alcohol's general availability could exacerbate the situation such that higher rates of these undesirable behaviors and conditions occur (Dull and Giacopassi, 1986, p. 519).

The investigators note that

. . . other researchers have found similar results. Room (1971) found that where there was no liquor by the drink, individuals tended to have either no alcohol or considerable quantities on hand at a given time. He speculated that this tended to encourage consumption of relatively greater quantities on a drinking occasion. Colón's (1982-83) research findings generally showed a significant and positive association between outlet frequency and rate of single vehicle fatalities. However, he also discovered that in reducing the number of outlets, a point of diminishing returns was reached where the relationship reversed itself. Colón hypothesized that the reversal of the association reflected the fact that where outlets were scarce, additional driving led to higher levels of vehicle fatalities. Popham, Schmidt, and de Lint (1976) found higher rates of arrest for drunkenness occurred where the outlet rates were lower in both Canada and in England.

In a review of the literature on studies dealing with alcohol availability, Popham, Schmidt, and de Lint (1981:584) [sic.; correct reference is Popham, Schmidt and de Lint, 1976, p. 584] concluded, "Summing up the evidence, it would seem clear that in the populations examined, variations in indicators of the prevalence of inebriety are not dependent on outlet frequency." (Dull and Giacopassi, 1986, p. 515).

The earlier-discussed research of Linsky and his colleagues (1986) is also relevant. Those researchers computed a proscriptivity index for each state in the U.S. based on the degree of legal restrictions on the sale or consumption of alcoholic beverages (number of on-premise liquor outlets per million population and degree to which on-premise sale of alcohol is restricted in hours or prohibited on Sundays and on other days of the week), the percentage of population living in dry areas, and the percentage of Mormons and Fundamentalists in the population. They found that there was less drinking in proscriptive states, but that the drinking that did occur tended to be more disruptive.

Colón and Cutter's (1983, p. 83) analysis of data from all 50 states and the District of Columbia revealed, "On-premise availability of alcohol was significantly and *inversely* associated with motor vehicle fatalities. This suggests that when on-premise outlets are fewer and more geographically spread out, the chances of drinking and driving are greater" (emphasis added). They (1983, p. 101) also found that "motor vehicle fatality rates for drivers in states with county-level prohibition were significantly greater than in nonprohibition states." Their finding that the average consumption of absolute alcohol is unrelated to highway fatalities "as well as those of Smart (1976), make it evident that the single distribution model of consumption cannot be extended to the province of highway safety" (Colón and Cutter, 1983, p. 88).

A methodologically sophisticated study of the effects of lifting a 58-year ban on alcohol advertising in Saskatchewan (Makowsky and Whitehead, 1991, p. 565) found that "advertising had no effect on total consumption." The researchers, proponents of the single distribution theory, concluded (p. 555) that "alcohol advertising is not a contributory force that influences the overall level of alcohol consumption. The place of advertising in the single distribution theory remains not proven, and the place of advertising as an instrument of public policy with respect to the prevention of alcohol-related damage remains in question."

These findings corroborate a study of the effects of print media advertising regulations in all states in the U.S. and of a beer advertising ban in Manitoba. The researchers (Ogborne and Smart, 1980, p. 295) found that states' "advertising restrictions were unrelated to per capita beer, wine or spirit consumption, to total per capita consumption or to alcoholism rate." They also found that beer consumption in Manitoba was unaffected by that province's ban on beer advertising and concluded (p. 293): "It is unlikely that restrictions on advertising will reduce consumption."

Smart and Cutler's (1976) study of a ban on all alcohol advertising in British Columbia similarly failed to detect any affect on consumption. Simon (1969) studied the affect of advertising on the sales of individual brands of spirits and concluded the size of advertising budgets did not contribute to the sales volume of individual brands. In their Canadian study, Bourgeois and Barnes (1979, p. 28) concluded that their research "produced little evidence to support the claim that the level of per-capita consumption of alcoholic beverage in Canada is influenced by the volume of advertising for these products."

In their review of research on the effects of advertising on alcohol consumption, Frankena et al. (1985) examined five studies. Only one (Comanor and Wilson, 1974) found a positive effect, that being for wine and spirits but not for malt liquor. However, the study has been criticized on methodological grounds (Grabowski, 1976). The other studies found no affect of alcohol advertising expenditures on the consumption of alcoholic beverages in general (Grabowski, 1976; Ashley et al., 1980), on the consumption of beer (Peles, 1971), or on the consumption of wine, spirits and malt liquor (Wilder, 1973-1974).

Four experimental studies were also reviewed by Frankena et al. (1985). In those experiments, subjects in New Zealand (Brown, 1978), Canada (Kohn et al., 1984; Kohn and Smart, 1984) and the United States (McCarthy and Ewing, 1983) were exposed to alcohol advertising and then their alcohol consumption was measured either then or at a later meal. Only one of the studies (Brown, 1978) found any influence of advertising on consumption. If advertising has any affect on consumption, it should be most easily detectable in an experimental design in which other variables are controlled and in which consumption is measured closely in time to the exposure to the persuasive message of advertising (Hanson, 1980, p. 11), although not everyone agrees with this view (Smart, 1988, p. 315).

Reviews of the literature (e.g., U.S. Department of Health and Human Services, 1990, pp. 211-212; Pittman and Lambert, 1978, p. 28; Moskowitz, 1989, p. 59; Whitehead, 1983; Frankena et al., 1985; Smart, 1982; 1988; Atkin, 1987, p. 273) suggest that if advertising has any affect at all on overall consumption levels, it is likely to be very small at best. Pittman and Lambert (1978, p. 28) conducted an extensive systematic review of the literature, concluding: "Nobody knows to what extent, if any, alcohol advertising contributes to alcohol consumption or alcohol abuse," and Pittman (1980, p. 18) later asserted that ". . . no scientific evidence exists that beverage alcohol advertising has any significant impact on the rate of alcohol abuse and alcoholism in American society." Connor (1980) observed, "The most striking conclusion about the relationship between advertising and the use and abuse of alcohol is that no firm conclusion can be drawn. . . ." On the basis of his extensive review,[16] (Smart, 1988, p. 314) concluded: "The evidence indicates that advertising bans do not reduce alcohol sales, total advertising expenditures have no reliable correlation with sales of alcoholic beverages, and that experimental studies typically show no effect of advertising on actual consumption" and "In general, the evidence indicates little impact of advertising on alcohol sales or drinking." Even the neo-prohibitionist Center for Science in the Public Interest "recognizes that the existing research does not demonstrate a causal connection between alcohol beverage advertising or marketing practices and increased alcohol consumption or alcohol abuse" (Federal Trade Commission, 1985, p. 1). On the basis of his extensive and detailed worldwide survey of research, Fisher (1993, p. 150) concluded that "advertising appears to have a very weak positive influence on consumption and no impact on experimentation with alcohol or abuse of it."

This is consistent with other research which has found advertising to have little or no impact on the overall consumption of consumer products (e.g., Schmalensee, 1972), although some research (e.g., Lambin, 1976) has found brand advertising to have a positive affect on a brand's share of the market. Importantly, some studies (e.g., Grabowski, 1976; Picconi and Olson, 1978) indicate that increased sales lead to increased advertising, not vice versa.

Evidence regarding the relationship between the price of alcoholic beverages and consumption is not so weak as that concerning most ideas proposed by control-of-consumption proponents. "Probably no [other] control factor has been so often studied as has price" (Smart, 1982, p. 233), and useful reviews of the research are presented by Ornstein (1980), Cook (1981), Smart (1982), Ornstein and Levy (1983), Babor (1985), Ashley and Rankin (1988).

However, much of the research has been seriously weakened by methodological problems:

Cook (1981) has discussed several common methodological problems with studies that examine the effects of price on consumption. First, the consumption measure is usually based upon wholesalers' reported sales which may be underreported to evade taxes. Also, this measure does not reflect illegal production of alcoholic beverages or purchases made outside of a region. These potential sources of tax evasion are likely to increase when there is a tax increase; thus, this consumption measure is likely to exaggerate any actual decline in consumption. Second, many econometric studies fail to control for socio-demographic differences and differences in other regulatory activity that may affect consumption. Finally, the price of a commodity tends to be influenced by the demand for the commodity; thus, conventional statistical analyses (i.e., ordinary least squares methods) produce biased estimates (Moskowitz, 1989, p. 58).

Experimental and quasi-experimental studies frequently lack comparison groups and/or are based on small numbers of subjects (Moskowitz, 1989, p. 59). Smart (1982, p. 235) points out:

Econometric analyses have not led to very clear conclusions about what type of price increase could be expected to lead to what decrease or change in alcohol consumption or problems. Demand for beverages may vary considerably across jurisdictions and in response to many factors other than price, including income. Heavy drinkers may not be much affected by price increases, and cheaper beverages can be substituted for the more expensive. In general, price seems to affect consumption but we cannot offer very definite suggestions to governments as to how to change prices to achieve any desired preventive effect without undesired losses.

Elasticity of demand[17] may not be constant (or may not even exist for some beverages (Lau, 1975; Lidman, 1976), localities, or sub-groups (such as gender, age, educational, religious, or drinking level) of the population (Vladeck and Weiss, 1975; Miller and Agnew, 1974; Kyvig, 1979, p. 25). On the basis of their careful study, Colón et al. (1981, p. 358) conclude:

The conception that alcohol behaves like many economic commodities (i.e., responsive to price, income, and availability conditions) is clearly an over-simplification. Socio-cultural variables, such as the cultural anomie of unintegrated groups and the role of churches in molding values toward alcohol, appear to play a major role in the demand for alcohol. Further, the relationship between extreme control measures and illicit supply suggests that the demand for alcohol across beverage types is inelastic, i.e., unresponsive to external control and manipulation.

Two availability dimensions were identified that shed light on the predictive role of this variable. Both forms of availability were significant predictors of consumption but not of alcoholism. It appears, then, that consumption in part is influenced by availability but the alcoholism rate is not. The degree of control over consumption is at best incomplete, since extreme controls appear to stimulate illicit supply.

Significantly, there is evidence (Parker and Harman, 1978; Colón, 1979, p. 94; Smart, 1977; Walsh and Walsh, 1970; Barsby and Marshall, 1977), that income is much more important than price in influencing consumption. However, lowering personal income to reduce alcohol consumption would not appear to be a palatable public policy.

Underlying minimum age legislation are the assumptions of American prohibitionism: alcohol consumption is sinful and dangerous; it results in problem behavior; and drinking in any degree is equally undesirable because moderate social drinking is the forerunner of chronic inebriation (Sterne et al., 1967). Naturally, young people, if not everyone, should be protected from alcohol, according to this view. However, following the repeal of the Eighteenth Amendment in 1933, prohibition efforts have largely been age-specific. "The youngest age group is . . . chosen as a symbolic gesture because of its political impotence and because . . . there are not major economic consequences . . ." (Mosher, 1980, p. 31). Minimum age requirements are often viewed as expressing and communicating society's view of appropriate (Grant, 1989, p. 72) or ideal conduct.

Moskowitz (1989, p. 60) points out, "Despite the long history of minimum age as an alcohol control policy and numerous opportunities to conduct natural experiments, there has been relatively little research on the effects of minimum age laws." Additionally, there is disagreement regarding the interpretation of that research. Ashley and Rankin (1988, p. 251) describe the data as "neither unflawed nor entirely consistent," while Single (1988, p. 338) asserts that "the findings regarding the impact of age restrictions are unequivocal" in identifying an inverse relationship between lower legal drinking age and alcohol consumption.

It can be stated unequivocally that the findings regarding age-specific prohibition are not unequivocal. For example, a study of a large sample of young people between the ages of 16 and 19 in Massachusetts and New York after Massachusetts raised its drinking age revealed that the average, self-reported daily alcohol consumption in Massachusetts did not decline in comparison with New York (Hingson et al., 1985). Comparison of college students attending schools in states that had maintained for a period of at least ten years a minimum drinking age of 21 with those in states that had similarly maintained minimum drinking ages below 21 revealed few differences in drinking problems (Engs and Hanson, 1986). Colón's (1984, p. 159) study of all 50 states and the District of Columbia found "a positive relationship between the purchase age and single-vehicle fatalities." Thus, he found single-vehicle fatalities to be more frequent in those states with high purchase ages.

Comparisons of drinking before and after the passage of raised minimum age legislation have generally revealed little impact upon behavior (Perkins and Berkowitz, 1985; Hanson and Hattauer, n.d. Davis, 1990; Williams et al., 1990). For example, a study that examined college students' drinking behavior before and after an increase in the minimum legal drinking age from 18 to 19 in New York State found the law to have no impact on under-age students' consumption rates, intoxication, drinking attitudes or drinking problems (Perkins and Berkowitz, 1985; 1989). These findings were corroborated by other researchers at a different college in the same state (Hanson and Hattauer, n.d.). A similar study at Texas A & M examined the impact of an increase in consumption or alcohol problems among under-age students. However, there was a significant increase among such students in attendance at events where alcohol was present. There were also significant increases in the frequency of their requests to legal-age students to provide alcohol and in their receipt of illicit alcohol from legal-age students (Mason et al., 1988).

A longitudinal study of the effect of a one-year increase of the drinking age in the province of Ontario found that it had a minimum effect on consumption among 18-and 19-year-old high school students and none among those who drank once a week or more (Vingilis and Smart, 1981). A similar study was conducted among college students in the State University System of Florida to examine their behavior before and after an increase in the drinking age from 19 to 21. While there was a general trend toward reduced consumption of alcohol after the change in law, alcohol-related problems increased significantly. Surveys at Arizona State University before and after that state raised the legal drinking age from 19 to 21 found no reduction in alcohol consumption (Williams et al., 1990). Finally, an examination of East Carolina University students' intentions regarding their behavior following passage of a new 21-year-age drinking law revealed that only 6% intended to stop drinking, 70% planned to change their drinking location, 21% expected to use a false or borrowed identification to obtain alcohol and 22% intended to use other drugs. Anecdotal statements by students indicated the belief of some that it "might be easier to hide a little pot in my room than a six pack of beer." (Lotterhos et al., 1988, p. 644).

Over the past four decades it has been demonstrated that the proportion of collegiate drinkers increases with age (Straus and Bacon, 1953; Wechsler and McFadden, 1979; Perkins and Berkowitz, 1987). However, in July of 1987 the minimum purchase age became 21 in all states. Because drinking tends to be highly valued among collegians and because it is now illegal for those under 21 to purchase alcohol, Engs and Hanson (1989) hypothesized that reactance motivation (Brehm and Brehm, 1981) would be stimulated among such students, leading more of them to drink. Their data from 3,375 students at 56 colleges across the country revealed that, after the legislation, significantly more under-age students drank compared to those of legal age. Thus, the increase in purchase age appears to have been not only ineffective but actually counter-productive, at least in the short run.

Mosher has pointed out that

these modern youthful-drinking laws and enforcement priorities contrast with trends in youthful-drinking patterns. In the abstract, one would predict that increasingly stringent controls on availability and emphasis on enforcement would lessen the actual amount of alcohol consumed. Indeed, for all the problems associated with national Prohibition, use did decline during that period. Such is not the case for youthful drinking. Statistics show that under-aged persons increased their use of alcohol steadily from the 1930s to the 1960s, when legislation to curtail sales was most active. Ironically, a plateau was reached both in the prevalence of teenage drinking and in legislative action to restrict availability to teenagers at approximately the same time (Mosher, 1980, p. 25).

Sterne and her colleagues (1967) concluded that minimum age laws not only fail in their intent but also produce very questionable unintended consequences:

1) The consumption of alcohol in automobiles is clearly undesirable, yet in denying the right of the older teenage to its public purchase and consumption, we unwittingly suggest this combination.
2) The practice of patterned evasion of stringent liquor laws is a poor introduction of youth to adult civic responsibility, suggesting adult roles which incorporate neither respect for nor conformity to the law.
3) As Prohibition amply demonstrated, liquor laws which do not meet with public acceptance provide illicit business opportunities. While taverns have not been found to be an important factor producing delinquency, a small minority of them capitalize on this opportunity for illicit business, catering to questionable entertainment and an outlet for drugs (Sterne et al., 1967, pp. 58-59).

Of course, minimum age laws are consistent with the new temperance movement in that they convey the message that alcohol is a dangerous drug to be avoided.

CONTROL AND SOCIO-CULTURAL VARIABLES TESTED HEAD-TO-HEAD: SOCIO-CULTURAL MODEL WINS

On the basis of his sophisticated nation-wide study of the United States, Colón (1979, p. 90) wrote, "Single distribution theorists contend that availability measures, including economic variables, determine consumption and, in turn, alcoholism. It is apparent that this linear model is untenable, since socio-demographic factors also enter into the determination of consumption levels. Socio-demographic variables not only contribute to consumption but are quantitatively more important."

Colón (1979, pp. 92-93) concludes that ". . . price is not an efficacious policy measure capable of controlling consumption" and that "whether the policy target is alcoholism or cirrhosis mortality, if a policy is based upon the assumption that consumption can be controlled by means of availability, including price, it rests on a foundation of sand," because that strategy is "totally untenable."

None of the other alcohol-control policies examined (the minimum legal purchase age, retail outlets per capita, on-premise drinking outlets per capita, state control of distribution, state taxes and county-level prohibition) had any significant influence on consumption (Colón, 1979, pp. 101-102).

Importantly, Colón (1979, pp. 93-94) found consumption to be insignificant in predicting alcoholism rates[18] and referred to Parker and Harman's (1978, p. 387) observation that "[h]eavy drinking may not equate to alcoholism on a 1:1 basis, and should be more carefully explored, e.g., body weight and diet intervene between consumption and cirrhosis as does pattern of drinking, whether steady or episodic."

Colón (1979, pp. 92-93) concludes: "The model of consumption that emerges from this study is a cross between socio-cultural variables and one economic variable--income. Ordering these variables on their strength suggests that the demand for absolute alcohol is determined primarily by socio-cultural factors, such as attitudes and the institutions that shape attitudes and norms." He explains: "Economic variables constitute limitations or constraints that are superimposed on the socio-cultural system. Given this double layering or ordering of factors influencing consumption, it is apparent that maximum leverage cannot be obtained in the second layer of economic variables." More recent studies (Rabow and Watts, 1982, p. 799; Heien and Pompelli, 1987, p. 455) also stress the importance of social variables in understanding alcohol abuse. In the words of Heien and Pompelli (1987, p. 455) their results "tend to highlight the importance of sociological factors and downplay the distribution of consumption variables."

SUMMARY AND CONCLUSION

In the early period of American life alcohol was widely used by men, women and children. However, its use was strongly controlled by social norms and abuse was infrequent. With the passage of time, with the occurrence of dramatic social change, and with the relaxation of social controls, abuse became more common in the early 1800s. A powerful temperance movement then arose which, during the 1830s, began calling not for the temperate or moderate use of alcohol but for nothing short of total abstinence.

After decades of propaganda by the WCTU and innumerable other temperance proselytizers, it is not surprising that many temperance beliefs and attitudes are now a part of our culture. The percentage of abstainers in the United States is, along with Ireland's, the highest among Western nations (Peele, 1989, p. 43). And in a 1987 Gallup Poll, 17% of the Americans interviewed said they would favor a law forbidding the sale of alcoholic beverages throughout the nation (Room, 1991, p.156). The neo-dry movement is a natural and understandable consequence of these facts.

The temperance movement appears to have had a strong appeal to authoritarian (Sinclair, 1962, ch. 2) and dogmatic (or closed-minded) persons. Such individuals tend to accept simplistic solutions to complex problems. They are intolerant of ambiguity and tend to see issues in dichotomized terms (Hanson, 1967, ch. 2). The temperance movement defined individuals as either abstainers or drunkards; abstinence was good, drinking was bad. Moderation or responsible use was rejected.[19] Alcohol itself was not defined as a substance that could be used or abused: it was a poison. Thus, ". . . either a person was *for* the movement or was *for* its enemies, the Wets (Bacon, 1970, p. 135, emphasis in original).

The new temperance proponents of today similarly reject ambiguity and uncertainty. Recall that the U.S. Department of Education (1988, p. 11 emphasis in original), for example, asserts, "Curricula which advocate '*responsible use*' of drugs should be rejected." It similarly warns against curricula that teach that "drugs themselves are neither good nor bad." And the complexity of real life must be denied so as not to send "conflicting messages." Recall that "another warning sign [of an unacceptable curriculum] is the 'some believe this . . . while others believe that' approach which avoids being 'judgmental' about drugs. Phrases like 'research is inconclusive' or 'not enough is known to make a judgment' about the effects of drugs are red flags." Similarly, the WCTU never feared being judgmental about alcohol or its effects and was also intolerant of mixed messages. Recall also that, like the WCTU, the Office for Substance Abuse Prevention (1987, p. 11) describes alcohol as a poison.

But the socio-cultural approach also arises out of the American past. While much of the positive early national experience with alcohol was later eclipsed, it was subsequently reinforced by the great migrations of Jews and Mediterranean peoples in the latter half of the last century and early part of this century. Millions of immigrants were from backgrounds in which the moderate use of alcohol was approved.

The temperance movement generally rejected immigrants and their use of alcohol,[20] and it is ironic that the neo-temperance movement of today rejects the lessons that can be learned from the successful use of alcohol by many of those same immigrant groups.

The new temperance movement rests heavily upon the Ledermann curve. Although "there is no known logical reason for the shape of the curve or the relationship between mean consumption and the proportion of heavy drinkers"

(Colón, 1979, pp. 11-12) and the empirical evidence is inadequate (Hilton and Clark, 1987, pp. 521-522), new temperance advocates continue to place their confidence in this model and its policy implications that drinking problems can be reduced by limiting the availability of alcohol through such measures as price increases, restricting sales to certain days or hours, mandating product warning labels and imposing age-specific prohibition.   They ignore variations in consumption among such significant categories as gender, age, race, religion, socio-economic status, ethnicity and occupation.   The control-of-consumption model "is neither a scientifically validated nor reliable model on which a society should base its primary prevention policy for the control of alcoholism and alcohol related damage" (Pittman, 1980, p. 59).

Importantly, even if control-of-consumption policies were to be effective in lowering mean per capita consumption, it is questionable whether or not drinking problems associated with heavy drinking would be reduced.[21]   Furthermore, lowering mean consumption among moderate drinkers would appear to be counterproductive for their health and longevity.   Thus, the simplistic solutions proposed by control-of-consumption proponents appear inadequate to deal with the complexities of the real world.   Ironically, to the extent that the new temperance movement can demonstrate its effectiveness in reducing the mean per capita consumption of alcohol, it may demonstrate its undesirability.

NOTES

1. In its early stages the temperance movement called for the temperate or moderate use of alcohol, although as early as 1800 there were isolated calls for abstinence (Plaut, 1967, p. 132). However, "it was not until the middle 1830s that total abstinence became the guiding principle of the temperance movement" (Asbury, 1950, p. 29). Many of the problems caused by industrialization, urbanization, massive immigration and social change were attributed to alcohol. As one temperance writer argued, "[the] unrestricted manufacture and sale of ardent spirits is almost the sole cause of all the suffering, the poverty, and the crime to be found in the country" (Temperance Writer, 1988, p. 16). Alcohol, "the good creature of God" had become "the demon rum" (Fingarette, 1988, p. 16; Rorabaugh, 1979, p. 219).

2. Hatred appears to have been characteristic of many Prohibitionists. For example, Billy Sunday, speaking metaphorically to alcohol, said "I hate you with a perfect hatred. I love to hate you" (Asbury, 1950, p. 144). Not only did they seek to train "haters of alcohol," but "Prohibitionists frequently . . . abused anyone who disagreed with them; indeed, derogatory and vituperative language became a trademark of the temperance crusade" (Isaac, 1965, p. 266).

One woman suggested that liquor law violators should be hung by the tongue beneath an airplane and carried over the United States. Another suggested that the government should distribute poison liquor through the bootleggers; she admitted that several hundred thousand Americans would die, but she thought that this cost was worth the proper enforcements of the dry law. Others wanted to deport all aliens, exclude wets from all churches, force bootleggers to go to church every Sunday, forbid drinkers to marry,

torture or whip or brand or sterilize or tatoo drinkers, place offenders in bottle-shaped cages in public squares, make them swallow two ounces of castor oil, and even execute the consumers of alcohol and their posterity to the fourth generation (Sinclair, 1962, p. 26); for other suggestions, see Tietsort, 1929, ch. 8).

3.   Cross-cultural analysis reveals: "The only 'prohibition' against alcohol consumption that seems to work in human society is that taken on *voluntarily* by the drinker himself . . ." (Marshall, 1979, p. 456, emphasis in original).

4.   The Volstead Act, passed by Congress to enforce the Eighteenth Amendment, attempted to prevent illegal trade in alcohol by means of fines and imprisonment (Kobler, 1973, p. 13).

5.   This view extends back to early history and is reflected in the teachings of Judaism and Christianity as well as in societies around the world. It was expressed by a pioneer in the socio-cultural approach, Robert Bales, when he wrote that ". . . it is necessary at the outset to avoid confusion between the degree to which alcohol is used in a given culture and the degree to which it creates problems in that culture . . . (Bales, 1946, p. 480).

6.   Ideally, children learn at home from good parental role models within a supportive family environment.

7.   While there is overwhelming consensus that Prohibition was a failure, there is not unanimity:

> Prohibition did not fail. On the contrary, it was a tremendous success. . . . [It] brought significant gains to society as a whole and made life more livable for many American families. . . . America prospered economically during the Prohibition period . . . it actually brought about a marked decrease in crime of all kinds . . . (A Methodist editor, 1970).

More recently, the federal Office for Substance Abuse Prevention (Resnik, 1990) has described Prohibition as a success in protecting Americans from the "dangerous drug of alcohol," as have some control-of-consumption writers (for example, Gross, 1983, p. 8; Single, 1988, p. 337). The WCTU, the Prohibition Party, the Anti-Saloon League (now known as the American Council on Alcohol Problems) and other groups continue to promote a return to temperance.

8.   Keller asserts:

> Fifty years after the end of prohibition, we are being advised to enact inhibition. Along with the scientists, the alcoholismists--with still mainly alcoholics in their ranks and leadership--are in full cry against alcohol. I have heard the foremost leader among them say, "If it hadn't been for alcohol, I would never have become an alcoholic." What he meant was, alcohol is the cause of alcoholism. And that is what many alcoholics would like to believe: that, of course, there was nothing wrong with them; that they were not primarily weak or deficient; that alcohol just happened to get the best of them. Once they stopped the alcohol, they were all right. So alcohol was the cause (Keller, 1985).

Control proponents appear frustrated that "the [alcohol beverage] industry does not acknowledge that alcohol is a problem in its own right . . ." (Ashley and Rankin, 1988, p. 239).

9. Many young adults under the age of 21 may resent being referred to as "kids" or as "children," the term used by the U.S. Department of Education (n.d., p. 3). Many parents may resent the implication that, by introducing their offspring to the enjoyment of alcohol with dinner or through the use of alcohol in their religious observances, they are "abusing" their charges.

10. Readers may be surprised to learn that the U.S. Department of Education considers alcohol to be an illicit drug. They may also be surprised to learn that it considers the use of alcohol in moderation to be generally unhealthful, given the overwhelming evidence to the contrary.

11. Pretending that there is scientific consensus on these controversial issues would appear to be more characteristic of propaganda than education for a democratic citizenry. The WCTU and other Prohibitionist groups similarly presented only those views, and those data, with which they agreed.

12. Writing in 1962, Sinclair (p. 41) pointed out: "Up to the present day, alcohol is still miscalled a poison in temperance publications, although it is no more than a mild sedative if taken in small quantities."

13. As indicated earlier, the WCTU similarly argued that alcohol can weaken the heart. However, it clearly specified its assertion that this may occur slowly "When alcohol is constantly [presumably it meant continually] used." OSAP provides no such qualifier.

14. An excellent description of the Ledermann model is provided by Miller and Agnew (1974).

15. A historian (Blocker, 1989, p. 156) has described the control-of-consumption approach as "a set of arguments dressed in modern social scientific garb" but which echo "arguments first made in the 1830's." Prendergast (1987, p. 26) makes a corroborative observation.

16. Smart (1988, p. 314), a control-of-consumption advocate, observes that " . . . some of the available reviews report data on only one side of the issue. For example, reviews by Katzper et al. (1978), Mosher and Wallace (1981) and Waterson (1983) leave out studies showing no effect of alcohol advertising. A recent review by the board of trustees of the American Medical Association (1986) quotes only a single controversial study showing that alcohol advertising affects youthful consumption but still suggests that a ban be undertaken." While Smart's point is significant, the Waterson review does not appear to be a good example of this bias.

17. "A commodity is said to have high price-elasticity if the demand reacts strongly to price changes, so that purchases go up steeply if prices go down, and purchases go down steeply if prices go up. Conversely, a product is said to be inelastic with respect to prices if purchases stay much the same when the price changes" (World Health Organization, 1980, p. 33).

18. On the basis of their study, Frankel and Whitehead (1985, p. 56) concluded that the prevalence of alcohol-related damage and the overall level of consumption are directly related. However, there is other evidence (for example, Peele, 1987, p. 68; Gusfield, 1974, p. 98) that the relationship between drinking problems and level of consumption is not consistent or clear.

19. "The temperance movement was not nearly as antidrunkard as it was opposed to those who claimed to be happy moderate drinkers, and the term *intemperate* was applied equally to habitual drunkards as to those who drank with meals" (Peele, 1989, p. 38,

emphasis in original).

20. It is no coincidence that legislation restricting the influx of immigration occurred during the height of the temperance movement's power. While some Catholics, political liberals (and presumably also some Germans and Jews) were pro-temperance (Timberlake, 1963, pp. 20-33; Bacon, 1970, p. 135), the largely anti-foreign, anti-Catholic, anti-German, anti-Semitic nature of the temperance movement has been widely documented. See, for example, Kobler (1973, pp. 168-169), Odegard (1928, pp. 24-35); Sinclair (1962, ch. 2 and pp. 119-126); Stivers 1983, p. 358); Hofstadter (1965, pp. 289-290).

21. Even if control-of-consumption policies were effective in reducing the problems caused by heavy drinkers, there remains the moral question posed by imposing the burdens of control policies on the lives of the vast majority of moderate drinkers who cause no problems and for whom alcohol improves their quality of life (Seixas, 1974, p. 20).

REFERENCES

Aaron, Paul and Musto, David. Temperance and Prohibition in America: An Historical Overview. In: Moore, Mark H., and Gerstein, Dean R. (eds.) *Alcohol and Public Policy: Beyond the Shadow of Prohibition.* Washington, DC: National Academy Press, 1981. pp. 127-180.

Alanko, Timo. Per Capita Consumption and rate of Heavy Use of Alcohol: On Evidence and Inference in the Single Distribution Debate. Paper presented at the Annual Alcohol Epidemiology Symposium of the Kettil Bruuh Society for Social and Epidemiological Research on Alcohol. Toronto, Ontario, May 30 - June 5, 1992.

American Council on Alcohol Problems. Introducing . . . American Council on Alcohol Problems. (leaflet) Bridgeton, MO: American Council on Alcohol Problems, n.d.

American Medical Association. Board of trustees report. Alcohol: advertising, counteradvertising, and depiction in the public media. *Journal of the American Medical Association,* 1986, *256,* 1485-1488.

Asbury, Herbert. *The Great Illusion: An Informal History of Prohibition.* New York: Doubleday & Co., 1950.

Ashley, Mary J. and Rankin, James G. A public health approach to the prevention of alcohol-related health problems. *Annual Review of Public Health,* 1988, *9,* 233-271.

Ashley, R., Granger, C. W. J., and Schmalensee, R. Advertising and aggregate consumption: An analysis of causality. *Econometrica,* 1980, *48,* 1149-1167.

Atkin, Charles K. Alcoholic-Beverage Advertising: Its Content and Impact. In: Holder, Harold D. and Mello, Nancy K. (eds.) *Control Issues in Alcohol Abuse Prevention: Strategies for States and Communities.* Greenwich, CT: JAI Press, 1987. pp. 267-303.

Babor, Thomas F. Alcohol, Economics and the Ecological Fallacy: Toward an Integration of Experimental and Quasi-Experimental Research. In: Single, Eric and Storm, T. (eds.) *Public Drinking and Public Policy.* Toronto, Ontario: Addiction Research Foundation, 1985. pp. 161-189.

Bacon, Margaret, and Jones, Mary B. *Teen-Age Drinking.* New York: Thomas Y. Crowell, 1968.

Bacon, Selden D. Meeting the Problem of Alcoholism in the United States. In: Whitney, Elizabeth D. (ed.) *World Dialogue on Alcohol and Drug Dependence* Boston: Beacon Press, 1970. pp. 134-145.

Bacon, Selden D. The role of law in meeting problems of alcohol and drug use and abuse. International Congress on Alcoholism and Drug Dependence, *Proceedings*, 20th, 1971, 162-172.

Bales, Robert F. Cultural differences in rates of alcoholism. *Quarterly Journal of Studies on Alcohol*, 1946, *6*, 480-499.

Barsby, Steve L. and Marshall, Gary L. Short-term consumption effects of a lower minimum alcohol-purchase age. *Journal of Studies on Alcohol*, 1977, *38*, 1665-1679.

Blocker, Jr., Jack S., *American Temperance Movements: Cycles of Reform.* Boston: Twayne, 1989.

Bourgeois, Jacques C., and Barnes, James G. Does advertising increase alcohol consumption? *Journal of Advertising Research*, 1979, *19*, 19-29.

Brehm, Sharon and Brehm, Jack W. *Psychological Reactance: A Theory of Freedom and Control.* New York: Academic Press, 1981.

Brown, R. A. Educating young people about alcohol use in New Zealand: Whose side are we on? *British Journal of Alcohol and Alcoholism*, 1978, *13*, 199-204.

Bruun, Kettil. *Drinking Behavior in Small Groups: An Experimental Study.* Helsinki, Finland: Finnish Foundation for Alcohol Studies, 1959.

Burnham, John C. New perspectives on the prohibition "experiment" of the 1920's. *Journal of Social History*, 1968, *2*, 51-68.

Chafetz, Morris E. Foreword. In: Fallding, Harold. *Drinking, Community and Civilization.* New Brunswick, NJ: Rutgers Center of Alcohol Studies, 1974. pp. xiii-xiv.

Christie, Nils. Goals, Ethics and Politics of Preventing Alcohol Problems. In: Room, Robin and Sheffield, Susan (eds.) *The Prevention of Alcohol Problems: Report of a Conference.* Sacramento, CA: Office of Alcoholism, Health and Welfare, 1974. pp. 2-11.

Colón, Israel. Alcohol Control Policies and Their Relation to Alcohol Consumption and Alcoholism. Unpublished Ph.D. dissertation, Brandeis University, 1979.

Colón, Israel. Alcohol availability and cirrhosis mortality rates by gender and race. *American Journal of Public Health*, 1981, *71*, 1325-1328.

Colón, Israel. The influence of state monopoly of alcohol distribution and the frequency of package stores on single motor vehicle fatalities. *American Journal of Drug and Alcohol Abuse*, 1982-1983, *9*, 315-331.

Colón, Israel. County-level prohibition and alcohol-related fatal motor vehicle accidents. *Journal of Safety Research*, 1983, *14*, 101-104.

Colón, Israel. The alcohol beverage purchase age and single-vehicle highway fatalities. *Journal of Safety Research*, 1984, *15*, 159-162.

Colón, Israel and Cutter, Henry S. G. The relationship of beer consumption and state alcohol and motor vehicle policies to fatal accidents. *Journal of Safety Research*, 1983, *14*, 83-89.

Colón, Israel, Cutter, Henry S. G., and Jones, Wyatt C. Alcohol control policies, alcohol consumption, and alcoholism. *American Journal of Drug and Alcohol Abuse*, 1981, *8*, 347-362.

Comanor, William, and Wilson, Thomas A. *Advertising and Market Power.* Cambridge, MA: Harvard University Press, 1974.

Connor, M. A. Advertising and alcohol consumption. *Bottom Line*, 1980, *4*, 12-13. Abstract #1311, *Journal of Studies on Alcohol*, 1981, *42*.

Conroy, D. W. Puritans and Taverns: Law and Popular Culture in Colonial

Massachusetts, 1630-1720. Paper presented at the Conference on the Social History of Alcohol: Drinking and Culture in Modern Society. Berkeley, CA, 1984. Cited by Prendergast, Michael L. A History of Alcohol Problem Prevention Efforts in the United States. In: Holder, Harold D. (ed.) *Control Issues in Alcohol Abuse Prevention: Strategies for States and Communities.* Greenwich, CT: JAI Press, 1987. p. 27.

Cook, Philip J. The effect of liquor taxes on drinking, cirrhosis and auto accidents. In: Moore, Mark H. and Gerstein, Dean R. (eds.) *Alcohol and Public Policy: Beyond the Shadow of Prohibition.* Washington, DC: National Academy Press, 1981. pp. 255-285.

Cowan, Richard. How the narcs created crack. *National Review,* 1986, *38,* 26-28, 30-31.

Davis, James E. Alcohol use among college students: Responses to raising the purchase age. *Journal of American College Health,* 1990, *38,* 263-269.

de Lint, Jan. Recent trends in Dutch drinking. A problem case for availability explanations. *Contemporary Drug Problems,* 1981, *10,* 179-192.

Drew, L. R. H. Road casualties - Australia 1952 to 1977: A reduced alcohol related problem. *Australian Journal of Alcoholism and Drug Dependency,* 1979, *5,* 122-123.

Duffy, John C. Comment on "The single distribution theory of alcohol consumption." *Journal of Studies on Alcohol,* 1978, *39,* 1648-1650.

Duffy, John C., and Cohen, G. R. Total alcohol consumption and excessive drinking. *British Journal of Addiction,* 1978, *73,* 259-264.

Dull, R. and Giacopassi, D. An assessment of the effects of alcohol ordinances on selected behaviors and conditions. *The Journal of Drug Issues,* 1986, *16,* 511-521.

Emerson, Haven. Prohibition and mortality and morbidity. *Annals of the American Academy of Political and Social Science,* 1932, *163,* 53-60.

Engelmann, Larry. *Intemperance: The Lost War Against Liquor.* New York: Free Press, 1979.

Engs, Ruth C., and Hanson, David J. Age-specific alcohol prohibition and college students' drinking problems. *Psychological Reports,* 1986, *59,* 979-984.

Engs, Ruth C., and Hanson, David J. Reactance theory: A test with collegiate drinking. *Psychological Reports,* 1989, *64,* 1083-1086.

Entine, A. D. The Relationship between the Number of Sales Outlets and the Consumption of Alcoholic Beverages in New York and other States. Albany, NY: New York State Moreland Commission of the Alcoholic Beverage Control Law, 1963. (Study Paper No. 2, October 21, 1963).

Everest, Allan S. *Rum Across the Border: The Prohibition Era in Northern New York.* Syracuse, NY: Syracuse University Press, 1978.

Ewing, John A., and Rouse, Beatrice A. Drinks, Drinkers, and Drinking. In: Ewing, John A., and Rouse, Beatrice A. (eds.) *Drinking: Alcohol in American Society - Issues and Current Research.* Chicago, IL: Nelson-Hall, 1976. pp. 5-30.

Fallding, Harold. *Drinking, Community and Civilization.* New Brunswick, NJ: Rutgers Center of Alcohol Studies, 1974.

Federal Trade Commission. *Recommendations of the Staff of the Federal Trade Commission: Omnibus Petition for Regulation of Unfair and Deceptive Alcoholic Beverage Advertising and Marketing Practices.* Washington, DC: Federal Trade Commission, 1985.

Fillmore, Kaye M. and Wittman, F. D. The effects of availability of alcohol on college student drinking: A trend study. *Contemporary Drug Problems,* 1982, *11,* 455-492.

Fingarette, Herbert. *Heavy Drinking.* Berkeley, CA: University of California Press, 1988.

Fisher, Joseph C. *Advertising, Alcohol Consumption, and Abuse: A Worldwide Survey.* Westport, CT: Greenwood Press, 1993.

Ford, Gene. *The Benefits of Moderate Drinking: Alcohol, Health and Society.* San Francisco, CA: Wine Appreciation Guild, 1988.

Frankel, B., and Whitehead, P. Effective Strategies for Prevention: Alcohol Problems and Public Health Policy. London, Ontario: University of Western Ontario, 1985. Cited by Moskowitz, Joel M. The primary prevention of alcohol problems: a critical review of the research literature. *Journal of Studies on Alcohol*, 1989, *50*, 58.

Frankena, M., Cohen, M., Daniel, T., Ehrlich, L., Greespun, N. and Kelman, D. Alcohol Advertising, Consumption and Abuse. In: Federal Trade Commission. *Recommendations of the Staff of the Federal Trade Commission: Omnibus Petition for Regulation of Unfair and Deceptive Alcoholic Beverage Marketing Practices, Dockett No. 209-46.* Washington, DC: Federal Trade Commission, 1985.

Georgia Department of Education. Quality Core Curriculum, Health and Safety, K-12. Atlanta, GA: Georgia Department of Education, n.d.

Gerstein, Dean R. Alcohol Use and Consequences. In: Moore, Mark H. and Gerstein, Dean R. (eds.) *Alcohol and Public Policy: Beyond the Shadow of Prohibition.* Washington, DC: National Academy Press, 1981. pp. 182-224.

Gliksman, Louis, and Rush, Brian R. Alcohol availability, alcohol consumption and alcohol-related damage. II. The role of sociodemographic variables. *Journal of Studies on Alcohol*, 1986, *47*, 11-18.

Gordis, Enoch. From science to social policy: An uncertain road. *Journal of Studies on Alcohol*, 1991, *52*, 101-109.

Grabowski, Henry G. The effects of advertising on the interindustry distribution of demand. *Explorations In Economic Research*, 1976, *3*, 21-75.

Grant, Marcus. Controlling Alcohol Abuse. In: Robinson, David, Mayard, Alan and Chester, Robert (eds.) *Controlling Legal Addictions.* New York: St. Martin;s Press, 1989. pp. 63-83.

Grant, Marcus and Ritson, Bruce. *Alcohol: The Prevention Debate.* New York: St. Martin's Press, 1983.

Graves, Karen L. Do Warning Labels on Alcoholic Beverages Make a Difference? A Comparison of the United States and Ontario, Canada between 1990 and 1991. Paper presented at the Annual Alcohol Epidemiology Symposium of the Kettil Bruun Society for Social and Epidemiological Research on Alcohol. Toronto, Ontario, May 30-June 5, 1992.

Gross, Leonard. *How Much is too Much?: The Effects of Social Drinking.* New York: Random House, 1983.

Gusfield, Joseph R. *Symbolic Crusade: Status Politics and the American Temperance Movement.* Urbana, IL: University of Illinois Press, 1963.

Gusfield, Joseph R. Status Conflicts and the Changing Ideologies of the American Temperance Movement. In: Pittman, David, J. and Snyder, Charles R. (eds.) *Society, Culture and Drinking Patterns.* New York: Wiley, 1962. pp. 101-120.

Gusfield, Joseph R. The Prevention of Alcohol Problems. In: Room, Robin and Sheffield, Susan (eds.) *The Prevention of Alcohol Problems: Report of a Conference* Sacramento, CA: Office of Alcoholism, Health and Welfare, 1974. pp. 90-113.

Hanson, David J. Dogmatism Among Specific Authoritarian and Non-Authoritarian

Response Types. Unpublished M.A. thesis, Syracuse University, 1967.

Hanson, David J.   Relationship between methods and findings in attitude-behavior research. *Psychology*, 1980, *17*, 11-13.

Hanson, David J. and Hattauer, Edward.   Effects of Legislated Drinking Norms on College Students' Behaviors. Potsdam, NY: Potsdam College of the State University of New York, unpublished paper, n.d.

Harford, Thomas C., Parker, Douglas A., Paulter, Charles, and Wolz, Michael. Relationship between the number of on-premise outlets and alcoholism. *Journal of Studies on Alcohol*, 1979, *40*, 1053-1057.

Heath, Dwight B.   Sociocultural Variants in Alcoholism. In: Pattison, E. Mansell and Kaufman, Edward (eds.) *Encyclopedic Handbook of Alcoholism*. New York: Gardner Press, 1982. pp. 426-440.

Heath, Dwight B.   A Decade of Development in the Anthropological Study of Alcohol Use: 1970-1980. In: Douglas, Mary (ed.) *Constructive Drinking: Perspectives on Drink from Anthropology*. Cambridge University Press, 1987. pp. 16-69.

Heath, Dwight B.   The new temperance movement: through the looking glass. *Drugs & Society*, 1989, *3*, 143-168.

Heien, Dale and Pompelli, Greg.   Stress, ethnic and distribution factors in a dichotomous response model of alcohol abuse. *Journal of Studies on Alcohol*, 1987, *48*, 450-455.

Herd, Denise.   Ideology, history and changing models of liver cirrhosis epidemiology. *British Journal of Addiction*, 1992, *87*, 1113-1126.

Hilton, Michael E. and Clark, Walter B.   Changes in American drinking patterns and problems, 1967-1984. *Journal of Studies on Alcohol*, 1987, *48*, 515-522.

Hingson, Ralph, Merrigan, Daniel, and Heeren, Timothy.   Effects of Massachusetts raising its legal drinking age from 18 to 20 on deaths from teenage homicide, suicide and nontraffic accidents. *Pediatric Clinics of North America*, 1985, *32*, 221-233.

Hofstadter, Richard.   *The Age of Reform: From Bryan to F.D.R.* New York: Vintage, 1965.

Holder, Harold D. and Blose, J. O.   Impact of changes in distilled spirits availability in apparent consumption: A time series analysis of liquor-by-the-drink. *British Journal of Addiction*, 1987, *82*, 623-631.

Honigmann, John J.   Dynamics of Drinking in an Austrian Village. In: Marshall, Mac (ed.) *Beliefs, Behaviors, & Alcoholic Beverages: A Cross-Cultural Survey*. Ann Arbor, MI: University of Michigan Press, 1979. pp. 414-428. Originally published in *Ethnology*, 1963, *2*, 157-169.

Hyman, Merton, Zimmerman, Marilyn, Gurioli, Carol, and Helrich, Alice.   *Drinkers, Drinking & Alcohol-Related Mortality & Hospitalization*. New Brunswick, NJ: Rutgers Center for Alcohol Studies, 1980.

Isaac, Paul E.   *Prohibition and Politics: Turbulent Decades in Tennessee 1885-1920*. Knoxville, TN: University of Tennessee Press, 1965.

Katzper, M., Ryback, R. and Hertzman, Marc.   Alcohol beverage advertisement and consumption. *Journal of Drug Issues*, 1978, *8*, 339-353.

Kaufman, E.   The relationship of alcoholism and alcohol abuse in the abuse of other drugs. *American Journal of Drug and Alcohol Abuse, 9*. Cited by Ford, Gene. *The Benefits of Moderate Drinking*. San Francisco, CA: Wine Appreciation Guild, 1988. pp. 137-138.

Keller, Mark.   Alcohol Problems and Policies. In: Kyvig, David E. (ed.) *Law, Alcohol, and Order*. Westport, CT: Greenwood Press, 1985. pp. 159-175.

Kerr, K. Austin. *Organized for Prohibition: A New History of the Anti-Saloon League*. New Haven, CT: Yale University Press, 1985.

Kobler, John. *Ardent Spirits: The Rise and Fall of Prohibition*. New York: G. P. Putnam's Sons, 1973.

Kohn, Paul M., and Smart, Reginald G. The impact of television advertising on alcohol consumption: An experiment. *Journal of Studies on Alcohol*, 1984, *45*, 295-301.

Kohn, Paul M., Smart, Reginald G. and Osborne, A. C. Effects of two kinds of alcohol advertising on subsequent consumption. *Journal of Advertising*, 1984, *48*, 34-40.

Kyvig, David E. *Repealing National Prohibition*. Chicago: University of Chicago Press, 1979.

Kyvig, David E. Sober Thoughts: Myths and Realities of National Prohibition after Fifty Years. In: Kyvig, David E. (ed.) *Law, Alcohol, and Order: Perspectives on National Prohibition*. Westport, CT: Greenwood Press, 1985. pp. 3-20.

Lambin, Jean-Jacques. *Advertising, Competition and Market Conduct in Oligapoly over Time*. Amsterdam, The Netherlands: North-Holland, 1976.

Lau, H. H. Cost of Alcoholic Beverages as a Determinant of Alcohol Consumption. In: Gibbins, R. J., Israel, Yedy, Kalant, Harold, Popham, Robert E., Schmidt, Wolfgang, and Smart, Reginald G. (eds.) *Research Advances in Alcohol and Drug Problems*. Vol. 2. New York: Wiley, 1975. pp. 211-245.

Lauderdale, Michael L. *An Analysis of the Control Theory of Alcoholism*. Denver, CO: Education Commission of the States, 1977.

Lazar, Irving and Ford, John. Untitled reaction of review panel. In: Lauderdale, Michael L. *An Analysis of the Control Theory of Alcoholism*. Denver, CO: Education Commission of the State, 1977. pp. 29-34.

Ledermann, Sully. *Alcoolisme, Alcoolisation: Données Scientifiques de Caractère Physiologique, Economique et Social*. Paris: Presses Universitaires de France, 1956.

Levine, Harry G. Temperance and Women in 19th-Century United States. In: Kalant, Oriana J. (ed.) *Alcohol and Drug Problems in Women: Research Advances in Alcohol and Drug Problems*. Vol. 5. New York: Plenum, 1980. pp. 25-67.

Levine, Harry G. The alcohol problem in America: From temperance to alcoholism. *British Journal of Addiction*, 1984, *79*, 109-119.

Lidman, R. M. Measuring spirits price elasticity in Canada and California: New findings. *Drinking and Drug Practices Surveyor*, 1976, No. 12, 9-13.

Linksy, A., Colby, J. and Strauss, M. Drinking norms and alcohol-related problems in the United States. *Journal of Studies on Alcohol*, 1986, *47*, 384-393.

Lotterhos, J. F., Glover, E. D., Holbert, D., and Barnes, R. C. Intentionality of college students regarding North Carolina's 21-year drinking age law. *International Journal of the Addictions*, *23*, Marcel Dekker Inc., NY, 1988, 629-647.

Maine State Department of Education. Leadership in Maine. (Poster) Augusta, ME: Maine State Department of Education, n.d.

Mäkelä, Klaus. Level of Consumption and Social Consequences of Drinking. In: Israel, Yedy, Glaser, Frederick B., Kalant, Harold, Popham, Robert E., Schmidt, Wolfgang, Smart, Reginald G. (eds.) *Research Advances in Alcohol and Drug Problems*, Volume 4. New York, Plenum Press, 1978. pp. 303-348.

Makowsky, Cheryl R. and Whitehead, Paul C. Advertising and alcohol sales: A legal impact study. *Journal of Studies on Alcohol*, 1991, *52*, 555-567.

Mandelbaum, David G. Alcohol and Culture. In: Marshall, Mac (ed.) *Beliefs,*

Behaviors, & Alcoholic Beverages: A Cross-Cultural Survey. Ann Arbor, MI: University of Michigan Press, 1979, pp. 14-30. Reprinted from *Current Anthropology*, 1965, *6*, 281-293.

Marshall, Mac. Conclusions. In: Marshall, Mac (ed.) *Beliefs, Behaviors, & Alcoholic Beverages: A Cross-Cultural Survey.* Ann Arbor, MI: University of Michigan Press, 1979. pp. 451-457.

Mason, Timothy, Myszka, Michael, and Winniford, Jennifer. Assessing the Impact of the 21-Year Old Drinking Age: The Texas A & M Study. Paper presented at the annual meeting of the New York State Sociological Association, Oswego, NY, October 7-8, 1988.

McCarthy, D. and Ewing, John. Alcohol consumption while viewing alcoholic beverage advertising. *International Journal of the Addictions*, 1983, *18*, 1011-1018.

Mecca, Andrew M. *Alcoholism in America: A Modern Perspective.* Belvedere, CA: California Health Research Foundation, 1980.

A Methodist editor. *The American Issue*, 1970 (January) quoted by Kobler, John. *Ardent Spirits.* New York: G. P. Putnam's Sons, 1973. p. 355.

Mielke, Dan and Holstedt, Peggy. *Oregon Alcohol and Drug Prevention Education (ADADE) Infused Lesson Guide, K12.* Salem, OR: Oregon Department of Education and Eastern Oregon State College, 1991.

Milgram, Gail G. *The Facts about Drinking.* Mount Vernon, NY: Consumers Union, 1990.

Miller, Guy H., and Agnew, Neil. The Ledermann model of alcohol consumption. *Quarterly Journal of Studies of Alcohol*, 1974, *35*, 877-898.

Miron, Jeffrey and Zweibel, Jeffrey. Alcohol consumption during prohibition. *American Economic Review: Papers & Proceedings*, 1991, *81*, 242-247.

Modell, Walter. Mass drug catastrophes and the roles of science and technology. *Science*, 1967, *156*, 346-351.

Moore, Mark H. Actually, prohibition was a success. *New York Times*, 1989 (October 16), p. A-21.

Morton, Mary B. *Criteria for the Development or Selection of Drug Prevention Curricula.* Atlanta, GA: Southeast Regional Center for Drug-Free Schools and Communities, 1990.

Mosher, James F. The History of Youthful-Drinking Laws: Implications for Current Policy. In: Wechsler, Henry (ed.) *Minimum-Drinking-Age Laws.* Lexington, MA: Lexington Books, 1980. pp. 11-38.

Mosher, James F. and Wallace, Lawrence M. Government regulations of alcohol advertising: Protecting industry profits versus promoting the public health. *Journal of Public Health Policy*, 1981, *2*, 333-353.

Moskowitz, Joel M. The primary prevention of alcohol problems: A critical review of the research literature. *Journal of Studies on Alcohol*, 1989, *50*, 54-88.

Mulford, Harold A. and Fitzgerald, J. L. Consequences of increasing off-premise wine outlets in Iowa. *British Journal of Addiction*, 1988, *83*, 1271-1279.

Mulford, Harold A., Ledolter, J., and Fitzgerald, J. L. Alcohol availability and consumption: Iowa sales data revisited. *Journal of Studies on Alcohol*, 1992, *53*, 487-494.

National Institute on Alcohol Abuse and Alcoholism. *Alcohol and Health: Third Special Report to the U.S. Congress.* Rockville, MD: National Institute on Alcohol Abuse and Alcoholism, 1978. DHEW Publication No. ADM 78-569.

National Temperance and Prohibition Council. National Leadership Specializing on Alcohol Issues. (Pamphlet) Evanston, IL: National Temperance and Prohibition Council, n.d.

National Temperance and Prohibition Council. 1991 Resolutions. Evanston, IL: National Temperance and Prohibition Council, 1991.

Nelli, Humbert S. American Syndicate Crime: A Legacy of Prohibition. In: Kyvig, David E. (ed.) *Law, Alcohol, and Order: Perspectives on National Prohibition*, 1985.

New York State Division of Alcoholism and Alcohol Abuse. *Alcohol: The Gateway Drug*. Albany, NY: New York State Division of Alcoholism and Alcohol Abuse, n.d.

New York State Division of Alcoholism and Alcohol Abuse. *A Prevention Plan for the 1990s*. Albany, NY: New York State Division of Alcoholism and Alcohol Abuse, n.d.a.

New York State Division of Alcoholism and Alcohol Abuse. Do You use Drugs? (Poster) Albany, NY: New York State Division of Alcoholism and Alcohol Abuse, n.d.c.

New York State Division of Alcoholism and Alcohol Abuse. Don't be fooled. (Poster) Albany, NY: New York State Division of Alcoholism and Alcohol Abuse, n.d.d.

Odegard, Peter H. *Pressure Politics: The Story of the Anti-Saloon League*. New York: Columbia University Press, 1928.

Office for Substance Abuse Prevention. *Be Smart! Don't Start! Just Say No!* Rockville, MD: Office for Substance Abuse Prevention, 1987. Department of Health and Human Services Publication No. ADM 87-1502.

Office for Substance Abuse Prevention. *What You Can Do About Drug Use in America*. Rockville, MD: Office for Substance Abuse and Prevention, 1988. Department of Health and Human Services Publication No. ADM 88-1572.

Office for Substance Abuse Prevention. *Drug-Free Communities: Turning Awareness into Action*. Rockville, MD: Office for Substance Abuse Prevention, 1989. Department of Health and Human Services Publication No. ADM 89-1562.

Ogborne, Alan C., and Smart, Reginald G. Will restrictions on alcohol advertising reduce alcohol consumption? *British Journal of Addiction*, 1980, *75*, 293-296.

Ornstein, Stanley I. Control of alcohol consumption through price increases. *Journal of Studies on Alcohol*, 1980, *41*, 807-818.

Ornstein, Stanley I. and Levy, D. Price and Income Elasticities of Demand for Alcoholic Beverages. In: Galanter, Marc (ed.) *Recent Advances in Alcoholism*. Vol. 1. New York: Plenum Press, 1983. pp. 303-345.

Parker, Douglas A., and Harman, Marsha S. The distribution of consumption model of prevention of alcohol problems. *Journal of Studies on Alcohol*, 1978, *39*, 377-399.

Parker, Douglas A. and Harman, Marsha S. A Critique of the Distribution of Consumption Model of Prevention. In: Harford, Thomas C. and Parker, Douglas A. (eds.) *Normative Approaches to the Prevention of Alcohol Abuse and Alcoholism*. Rockville, MD: National Institute on Alcohol Abuse and Alcoholism, 1979. pp. 67-88.

Peele, Stanton. The limitations of control-of-supply models for explaining and preventing alcoholism and drug addiction. *Journal of Studies on Alcohol*, 1987, *48*, 61-77.

Peele, Stanton. *Diseasing of America: Addiction Treatment out of Control*. Lexington, MA: Lexington Books, 1989.

Peles, Yoram. Rates of amortization of advertising expenditures. *Journal of Political Economy*, 1971, *79*, 1032-1058.

Perkins, H. Wesley and Berkowitz, Alan D. College Students' Attitudinal and Behavioral Responses to a Drinking-Age Law Change: Stability and Contradiction in the Campus Setting. Paper presented at the annual meeting of the New York State Sociological Association, Rochester, NY, October 18-19, 1985.

Perkins, H. Wesley and Berkowitz, Alan D. Stability and Contradiction in College Students' Drinking Following a Drinking Law Change. Paper presented at the joint meeting of the American College Personnel Association and the National Association of Student Personnel Administrators, Chicago. March 15-18, 1987.

Perkins, H. Wesley and Berkowitz, Alan D. Stability and contradiction in college students' drinking following a drinking-age law change. *Journal of Alcohol and Drug Education*, 1989, *35*, 60-77.

Picconi, M. I., and Olson, C. L. Advertising decision rules in a multibrand environment: optional control theory and evidence. *Journal of Marketing Research*, 1978, *15*, 87-92.

Pittman, David J. *Primary Prevention of Alcohol Abuse and Alcoholism: An Evaluation of the Control of Consumption Policy.* St. Louis, MO: Washington University, Social Science Institute, 1980.

Pittman, David J. The New Temperance Movement. In: Pittman, David J. and White, Helene R. (eds.) *Society, Culture, and Drinking Patterns Reexamined.* New Brunswick, NJ: Rutgers Center of Alcohol Studies, 1991. pp. 775-790.

Pittman, David J. and Lambert, M. Dow. *Alcohol, Alcoholism & Advertising.* St. Louis, MO: Washington University, Social Science Institute, 1978.

Plaut, Thomas F. A. *Alcohol Problems: A Report to the Nation by the Cooperative Commission on the Study of Alcoholism.* New York: Oxford University Press, 1967.

Popham, Robert E. The Social History of the Tavern. In: Israel, Yedy, Glaser, Frederick B., Kalant, Harold, Popham, Robert E., Schmidt, Wolfgang, and Smart, Reginald G. (eds.) *Research Advances in Alcohol and Drug Problems.* Vol. 4. New York: Plenum, 1978. pp. 225-302.

Popham, Robert, Schmidt, Wolgang, and de Lint, Jan. The Effects of Legal Restraint on Drinking. In: Kissin, Benjamin and Begleiter, Henri (eds.) *Social Aspects of Alcoholism.* New York: Plenum Press, Vol. 4, 1976. pp. 579-625.

Popham, Robert, Schmidt, Wolfgang, and de Lint, Jan. Government Control Measures to Prevent Hazardous Drinking. In: Ewing, John A., and Rouse, Beatrice A. (eds.) *Drinking: Alcohol in American Society. Issues and Current Research.* Chicago: Nelson-Hall, 1978. pp. 239-266.

Prendergast, Michael L. A History of Alcohol Problem Prevention Efforts in the United States. In: Holder, Harold D. (ed.) *Control Issues in Alcohol Abuse Prevention: Strategies for States and Communities.* Greenwich, CT: JAI Press, 1987. pp. 25-52.

Rabow, Jerome, and Watts, Ronald K. Alcohol availability, alcoholic beverage sales and alcohol-related problems. *Journal of Studies on Alcohol*, 1982, *43*, 767-801.

Resnick, Hank. *Youth and Drugs: Society's Mixed Messages.* Rockville, MD: Office for Substance Abuse Prevention, 1990.

Room, Robin. Drinking in the Rural South: Some Comparisons in a National Sample. In Ewing, John A. and Rouse, Beatrice (eds.) *Law and Drinking Behavior.* Chapel Hill, NC: University of North Carolina, Center for Alcohol Studies, 1971. pp. 29-108.

Room, Robin. Cultural Changes in Drinking and Trends in Alcohol Problems Indicators: Recent U.S. Experience. In: Clark, Walter B. and Hilton, Michael E. (eds.) *Alcohol in America: Drinking Practices and Problems.* Albany, NY: State University of New York Press, 1991. pp. 149-162.

Rorabaugh, William. *The Alcoholic Republic.* New York: Oxford University Press, 1979.

Rose, Peter. If it feels good, it must be bad. *Fortune,* 1991. *122,* pp. 91, 92, 96, 100, 104, and 108.

Rush, Brian R., Gliksman, Louis, and Brook, Robert. Alcohol availability, alcohol consumption and alcohol-related damage. I. The distribution of consumption model. *Journal of Studies on Alcohol,* 1986, *47,* 1-10.

Sadava, S. W. Problem behavior theory and consumption and consequences of alcohol use. *Journal of Studies on Alcohol,* 1985, *46,* 392-397.

Schmalensee, Richard. *The Economics of Advertising.* Amsterdam, The Netherlands: North-Holland, 1972.

Schut, Jacob, File, Karen, and Wohlmuth, Theodora. Alcohol use by narcotic addicts in methadone maintenance treatment. *Quarterly Journal of Studies on Alcohol,* 1973, *34,* 1356-1359.

Seixas, Frank A. Goals, Ethics and Politics of Prevention of Alcohol Problems. In: Room, Robin and Sheffield, Susan (eds.) *The Prevention of Alcohol Problems: Report of a Conference.* Sacramento, CA: Office of Alcoholism, Health and Welfare, 1974. pp. 12-24.

Simon, Julian L. The economic effects of state monopoly of packaged-liquor retailing. *Journal of Political Economy,* 1966, *74,* 188-194.

Simon, Julian L. The effect of advertising on liquor brand sales. *Journal of Marketing Research,* 1969, *6,* 301-313.

Sinclair, Andrew. *Prohibition: The Era of Excess.* Boston: Little, Brown and Co., 1962.

Single, Eric W. The availability theory of alcohol-related problems. In: Chaudron, C. Douglas and Wilkinson, D. Adrian (eds.) *Theories on Alcoholism.* Toronto, Canada: Addiction Research Foundation, 1988. pp. 325-351.

Skog, Ole-Jørgen. Less alcohol--fewer alcoholics? *The Drinking and Drug Practices Surveyor,* 1973, No. 7, 7-13.

Smart, Reginald G. Per capita alcohol consumption, liver cirrhosis rates and drinking and driving. *Journal of Safety Research,* 1976, *8,* 112-115.

Smart, Reginald G. The Impact of Prevention Measures: An Examination of Research Findings. In: Institute of Medicine. *Legislative Approaches to Prevention of Alcohol-Related Problems: An Inter-American Workshop-Proceedings.* Washington, DC: National Academy Press, 1982. pp. 224-246.

Smart, Reginald G. The relationship of availability of alcoholic beverages to per capita consumption and alcoholism rates. *Journal of Studies on Alcohol,* 1977, *38,* 891-896.

Smart, Reginald G. Does alcohol advertising affect overall consumption? A review of empirical studies. *Journal of Studies on Alcohol,* 1988, *49,* 314-323.

Smart, Reginald G., and Cutler, R. E. The alcohol advertising ban in British Columbia: Problems and effects on beverage consumption. *British Journal of Addiction,* 1976, *71,* 13-21.

Smith, C. J. The wrath of grapes: The health-related implications of changing American drinking practices. *Area,* 1985, 97-108.

State Education Department of New York. *A Framework for Prevention.* Albany, NY: State Education Department, n.d.

Sterne, Muriel W., Pittman, David J. and Coe, Thomas. Teenagers, Drinking and the Law: Study of Arrest Trends for Alcohol-Related Offenses. In: Pittman, David J. (ed.) *Alcoholism*. New York: Harper and Row, 1967. pp. 55-56.

Stivers, Richard. Religion and Alcoholism. In: Kissin, Benjamin and Begleiter, Henri (eds.) *The Pathogenesis of Alcoholism: Psychosocial Factors*. New York: Plenum, 1983. pp. 341-364.

Straus, Robert and Bacon, Selden D. *Drinking in College*. New Haven, CT: Yale University Press, 1953.

Strayton, W. H. Our experiment in national Prohibition. What progress has it made? *Annals of the American Academy of Political and Social Science*, 1923, *109*, 26-38.

Sulkunen, P. Drinking Patterns and the Level of Alcohol Consumption: An International Overview. In: Gibbins, R. J., Israel, Yedy, Kalant, Harold, Popham, Robert E., Schmidt, Wolfgang, and Smart, Reginald G. (eds.) *Research Advances in Alcohol and Drug Problems*, Volume 3. New York: John Wiley & Sons, 1976. pp. 223-281.

Temperance Writer cited by Bernard, Joel. From the Fast Day Sermon to the Temperance Address: The Psychic Origins of a Social Movement. Paper presented at Conference on the Social History of Alcohol. Berkeley, CA, 1984. Cited by Fingarette, Herbert. *Heavy Drinking*. Berkeley, CA: University of California Press, 1988. p. 16.

Tietsort, Francis J. (ed.) *Temperance - or Prohibition?* New York: New York American, 1929.

Timberlake, James H. *Prohibition and the Progressive Movements: 1900-1920*. Cambridge, MA: Harvard University Press, 1963.

U.S. Department of Education. *Drug Prevention Curricula: A Guide to Selection and Implementation*. Washington, DC: U.S. Department of Education, 1988.

U.S. Department of Education. *Growing Up Drug Free: A Parent's Guide to Prevention*. Washington, DC: U.S. Department of Education, n.d.

U.S. Department of Education. *Drug Prevention Education*. Washington, DC: Department of Education, 1988.

U.S. Department of Health and Human Services. *Alcohol and Health: Seventh Special Report to the U.S. Congress on Alcohol and Health From the Secretary of Health and Human Services*. Rockville, MD: U.S. Department of Health and Human Services, 1990.

Vingilis, E. and Smart, Reginald G. Effects of raising the legal drinking age in Ontario. *British Journal of Addiction*, 1981, *76*, 415-424.

Vladeck, Bruce C., and Weiss, R. J. Policy alternatives for alcohol control. *American Journal of Public Health*, 1975, *65*, 1340-1342.

Wallack, M. J. The Advertising Debate. In: Grant, Marcus and Ritson, Bruce (eds.) *Alcohol and the Prevention Debate*. New York: St. Martin's Press, 1983. pp. 105-118.

Walsh, B. M., and Walsh, D. Economic aspects of alcohol consumption in the Republic of Ireland. *Economic and Social Review*, Dublin, 1970, *2*, 115-138.

Warburton, Clark. *The Economic Results of Prohibition*. New York: Columbia University Press, 1932. Reprinted by AMS Press, New York, 1968.

Washburne, Chander. *Primitive Drinking: A Study of the Uses and Functions of Alcohol in Preliterate Societies*. New York: College and University Press, 1961.

Waterson, M. J. The Advertising Debate. In: Grant, Marcus and Ritson, B. (eds.) *Alcohol and the Prevention Debate*. New York: St. Martin's Press, 1983. pp. 105-

118.

Wechsler, Henry and McFadden, Mary. Drinking among college students in New England. *Journal of Studies on Alcohol*, 1979, *40*, 969-996.

Whitehead, P. Is Advertising Effective? Implications for Public Health Policy. In: Rush, Brian and Ogbourne, Allan C. (eds.) *Evaluation Research in the Canadian Addictions Field*. Ottawa: Health and Welfare Canada, 1983. pp. 136-164.

Whitten, David N. Wine and health: A physician's view. *Wines & Vines*, 1988. pp. 32-33.

Wilder, R. P. Advertising and inter-industry competition: Testing a Galbraithian hypothesis. *Journal of Industrial Economics,* 1973-1974, *22,* 215-226.

Wilkinson, Rupert. *The Prevention of Drinking Problems*. New York: Oxford University Press, 1970.

Williams, Frank G., Kirkman-Liff, Bradford L., and Szivek, Pamela H. College student drinking behaviors before and after changes in state policy. *Journal of Alcohol and Drug Education*, 1990, *35*, 12-25.

World Health Organization. *Problems Related to Alcohol Consumption*. Geneva, Switzerland: World Health Organization, 1980.

Zimmer, Lynn and Morgan, John P. Prohibition's Costs - Always Too High? Paper presented at the annual meetings of the Kettil Bruun Society for Social and Epidemiological Research on Alcohol. Toronto, Ontario: May 30 - June 5, 1992.

Zinberg, Norman E., and Fraser, Kathleen M. The Role of the Social Setting in the Prevention and Treatment of Alcoholism. In: Mendelson, Jack H. and Mello, Nancy K. (eds.) *The Diagnosis and Treatment of Alcoholism*. New York: McGraw-Hill, second edition, 1985. pp. 457-483.

4

Summary and Recommendations

Beverage alcohol has always played a valuable role in enhancing the quality of human life. Alcohol causes few problems in the majority of societies throughout the world, although in some, drinking problems are seen as a cause of concern. Drinking abuse is least likely to occur in societies in which moderate drinking is encouraged and abusive drinking is sanctioned, in which there is consensus about what constitutes appropriate drinking behavior, in which people learn appropriate drinking from an early age, in which there is low social pressure to drink and in which emotionalism does not surround the subject of alcohol. While Prohibition has failed in the United States and in every other modern society, the prohibitionist desire is expressed today in the controversial control-of-consumption approach, which seeks to increase abstinence and to reduce the mean per capita consumption of alcohol. This is promoted as public policy in spite of overwhelming scientific evidence that the moderate consumption of alcohol is correlated with a lower incidence of heart and other diseases in particular and with greater longevity in general. On the other hand, there is little evidence that reducing the average consumption of alcohol reduces the incidence of drinking problems or that control-of-consumption policies are effective in reducing either average consumption or drinking problems. But even if they could ever be made effective in reducing average consumption among drinkers, that success would probably lead to an increase in heart and other diseases and a shorter life span for light and moderate drinkers without any offsetting positive effect for the minority of drinkers who consume heavily. This is clearly an unacceptable tradeoff. Therefore, understandings based on the cross-cultural and scientific evidence yield recommendations that the current control-of-consumption attack upon alcohol should be ended; that all attempts to stigmatize alcohol as a "dirty drug," as a poison, as inherently harmful or as a substance to be abhorred and shunned should be ended; that governmental agencies formulate and implement policies that incorporate the concept of moderate or responsible drinking along with the choice of abstinence; that systematic efforts be made to clarify and emphasize the distinctions between acceptable and unacceptable drinking; that unacceptable drinking behaviors be strongly sanctioned, both legally and socially; that parents be permitted to serve alcohol to their offspring of any age, not only at home, but in restaurants, parks and other locations under their direct control and supervision; and that educational efforts encourage moderate use of alcohol among those who choose to drink.

Alcohol has been in continuous use by peoples around the world throughout history. Long associated with religion, this highly valued beverage has also nourished the physical body with important nutrients and calories. Not only providing relief from pain, it has played an important medicinal and therapeutic role in human life. An important thirst quencher and safe alternative to polluted water, alcohol has also played an important role in enhancing the enjoyment and quality of life.

ALCOHOL USE AND ABUSE REFLECTS SOCIETY

While most societies around the world today consider alcohol to be a valuable part of life, a few reject it as threatening and unacceptable. But even among that vast majority accepting and using alcohol, it is not defined and perceived uniformly. Norms and cultural expectations affect not only how people react to the idea of alcohol and to people who use it, but also heavily influence how it affects those who consume it (Bacon and Jones, 1968, p. 12; MacAndrew and Edgerton, 1969; Mandelbaum, 1979, p. 15).

People learn what their society believes about alcohol and, acting in conformity with these beliefs, their behaviors become a self-fulfilling prophesy (MacAndrew and Edgerton, 1969, p. 88). Experimental evidence (e.g., Marlatt and Rohsenow, 1981) demonstrates that people tend to act in conformity to their beliefs about what they are drinking. For example, men who believed they were drinking vodka (but were only drinking tonic water) become more aggressive. However, when they were drinking vodka but thought it was only tonic water, they did not become more aggressive. And similar results are found for feelings of anxiety and sexuality.

"A major finding, in cross-cultural perspective, is that alcohol-related problems are really rare, even in many societies where drinking is customary, and drunkenness is commonplace" (Heath, 1987, pp. 18-19). Anthropologists generally agree that "most societies that use alcohol are virtually free of alcohol-related troubles" (Heath, 1987, p. 36) and "few have anything that might be called 'alcoholism' or even frequent 'drinking problems,' even when drinking and drunkenness are common" (Heath, 1987, p. 34). Marshall (1979, p. 452) observes that moralistic attitudes toward alcohol tend to be associated with its abuse.

It should be clear that attitudes, beliefs and social norms profoundly influence the way in which people behave when they drink as well as the resulting incidence of drinking problems (or lack of problems) in their group or society.

THE AMERICAN EXPERIENCE WITH ALCOHOL

During the first century and a half of American life, alcohol was widely and heavily used. Small children drank beer, wine and cider with their parents, and regular use was seen as healthful for everyone (Asbury, 1950, pp. 3-4; Sinclair, 1962, pp. 36-37; Popham, 1978, pp. 267-277).

By the time of the Revolutionary War there was an increased acceptance of intoxication and an increase in alcohol problems. During the social upheaval following the war, social control over drinking declined and it increasingly became an individualistic behavior (Peele, 1989, p. 69; Rorabaugh, 1979, p. 125; also Levine, 1980, p. 32; Fallding, 1974, p. 26). It became segregated by gender and age, which encouraged excessive consumption and drinking problems.

With the passage of time and the improvement of social conditions, especially as the West was settled, drunkenness became less acceptable (Zinberg and Fraser, 1985, p. 467). Stronger family life and the influx of immigrants from Europe also contributed to more moderate drinking patterns and behaviors (Asbury, 1950, p. 1). Ironically, while drinking behaviors were moderating, there was increased concern that drinking was not consistent with industrial development and efficiency, and prohibitionism became an increasingly powerful force (Strayton, 1923, p. 34).

Prohibitionist groups provided innumerable abstinence speakers, books, pamphlets, posters, curricular materials, sermons for clergy, and other abstinence materials. Much of this, presented as "scientific," was patently false propaganda (Goldberg, 1985, pp. 23-24). Importantly, prohibitionists tended to cast all issues in black and white terms: either one was an abstainer or was (or would become) a drunkard. The concept of moderation was adamantly rejected (Kobler, 1973, p. 140).

The political success of prohibitionists lead to the "great experiment" of Prohibition (1920-1933), which is widely recognized as a failure. On the one hand it failed to produce abstinence, while on the other it led to the extensive production of dangerous boot-leg alcohol, the rise of organized crime empires, widespread political corruption and general contempt for law (Engelmann, 1979; Kobler, 1973, ch. 10-13; Sinclair, 1962, ch. 9-15; Asbury, 1950, ch. 9-14; Everest, 1978; Grant and Ritson, 1983, p. 21). Thus, Prohibition was ineffective and counter-productive, just as it proved to be elsewhere around the world (Marshall, 1979, p. 456; Heath, 1987, p. 46; Ewing and Rouse, 1976).

An important counter-productive effect of Prohibition was that it encouraged the rapid consumption of high-proof drinks in secretive, non-socially regulated and controlled ways. When people took the trouble to go to a speakeasy, they didn't do so in order to have a leisurely beer but in order to get drunk. Removing alcohol from the social controls of everyday society both eliminated the growth of moderate drinking practices that had been increasing before Prohibition and increased drinking problems (Zinberg and Fraser, 1985).

ALTERNATIVE APPROACHES TO REDUCING ALCOHOL PROBLEMS

Approaches to reducing drinking problems can be generally categorized socio-culturally oriented or control-of-consumption oriented. The socio-cultural model tends to assume that

1) It is the misuse of alcohol, not alcohol itself, that is the source of drinking problems.
2) It is important to distinguish between drinking and alcohol abuse.
3) The misuse of alcohol can be reduced by educating individuals to make one of two decisions:
   - one decision is to abstain;
   - the other decision is to drink responsibly.
4) Because many individuals will choose to drink alcohol, it is important that societal norms regarding what is acceptable and unacceptable behavior for those who choose to drink be clear and unambiguous.
5) People who are going to drink as adults should gradually learn how to drink.

On the other hand, the control-of-consumption model tends to assume that

1) The substance of alcohol is the necessary and sufficient cause of all drinking problems.
2) The availability of alcohol determines the extent to which it will be consumed.
3) The quantity of alcohol consumed (rather than the manner in which it is consumed, the purpose for which it is consumed, the social context in which it is consumed, etc.) determines the extent of drinking problems.
4) Educational efforts should be directed toward stressing the problems that alcohol consumption can cause and encouraging abstinence.

Earlier control-of-consumption advocates called for total prohibition. Recognizing political reality, current advocates now more typically call for a diversity of measures designed to reduce rather than prohibit consumption. These include such policies as imposing higher taxes on alcoholic beverages, limiting or reducing the number of sales outlets, further restricting the permissible location for sales outlets, limiting the alcoholic content of beverages, prohibiting or limiting the advertising of alcohol, requiring the use of warning messages with all advertisements and on all beverage containers, requiring the display of warning signs in establishments that sell or serve alcoholic beverages, limiting the days or hours during which alcohol can be sold, increasing server liability for subsequent problems associated with the use of alcohol, limiting the sale of alcohol to people of specific ages, decreasing the legal alcohol blood content level for driving vehicles, and eliminating the tax deductibility of alcohol as a business expense.

The control-of-consumption approach assumes that the problem is alcohol while the socio-cultural approach assumes that the misuse of alcohol is the problem.   Hence, control-of-consumption policies attempt to prevent or discourage people from consuming alcohol, while socio-cultural policies attempt to prevent people from using alcohol irresponsibly.

A major thrust of control-of-consumption proponents is to reject the concept of responsible drinking and to stigmatize alcohol by associating it with illicit drugs. Linguistically, this is accomplished by insistence on referring to "alcohol and other drugs." Frequently it is accomplished by discussing alcohol in the same paragraph with crack cocaine and other illegal drugs. Another approach is to describe alcohol as harmful to the body, as "a mind-altering drug needing consideration with all other mind-altering drugs" (Maine State Department of Education, n.d.), or as leading to the use of illicit drugs. An even more blatant effort to stigmatize beverage alcohol is illustrated by Ernest Nobel, former Director of the National Institute on Alcoholism and Alcohol Abuse, in his assertion that "Alcohol is the dirtiest drug we have" and that it is more dangerous than heroin or LSD (Gross, 1983, p. 19).

Control-of-consumption publications often present alcohol as a "gateway drug" that will lead people into illicit drug use. The "evidence" is that most people who are involved with illicit drugs drank alcohol first. Of course, most illicit drug users also earlier drank orange juice, ate hamburgers and chewed gum.

The control-of-consumption model (sometimes called the control, the control of production, the availability, the new temperance, the neo-Prohibitionist and the neo-dry model) is frequently referred to as the single distribution model.

The single distribution model is based on the assumption that knowledge of the mean per capita consumption of absolute alcohol permits prediction of the proportion of heavy drinkers. It is asserted that if the mean consumption increases, the proportion of heavy drinkers will increase (Smith, 1985, p. 103). The assumption underlying the single distribution theory is that specific human behaviors invariably conform to a simple mathematical distribution in any and every population, a speculation that is demonstrably incorrect (Duffy, 1978, pp. 1649-1650; Pittman, 1980, p. 44). Yet regardless of both logical (Alanko, 1992, pp. 3-5) and empirical evidence (Hilton and Clark, 1987, pp. 521-522; Engs and Hanson, 1994, pp. 521-522; Engs and Hanson, 1994) to the contrary, control-of-consumption advocates still cling to their assumption that a change in the mean per capita consumption of alcohol will always lead to a very precise and predictable change in consumption among heavy drinkers.

In concerning themselves almost exclusively with the level of alcohol consumption, control-of-consumption advocates typically ignore other important variables related to drinking problems, such as diet, body weight, drinking patterns and culture. Perhaps reflecting cultural factors, there appears to be a strong inverse relationship between a country's level of alcohol consumption and its rate of drinking problems (Peele, 1989, p. 67). Others have reported that the incidence of cirrhosis is often poorly correlated with consumption level (de Lint, 1981; Sulkunen, 1976), as are other drinking problems (Peele, 1989, p. 68; Mäkelä, 1978, p. 344; Bruun, 1959).

A major issue is whether or not reducing mean per capita consumption would result in undesirable unanticipated consequences. Would it reduce one set of problems while increasing another? For example, would it result in a change from steady to episodic consumption with a higher quantity consumed per occasion? Keeping in mind the apparent health benefits and contribution to longevity of the moderate consumption of alcohol compared to either abstinence or heavy drinking, would it lead to fewer problems for formerly heavy drinkers but to increased health problems and reduced longevity for previously moderate and light drinkers?

After conducting a sophisticated nation-wide study of the United States, Colón (1979, p. 90) concluded that socio-demographic factors were much more important that availability factors. None of the control policies he examined (price, minimum legal purchase age, retail outlets per capita, on-premise drinking outlets per capita, state control of distribution, state taxes, and county-level prohibition) had any significant influence on consumption (Colón, 1979, pp. 90 and 101-102). Other studies (Rabow and Watts, 1982, p. 799; Heien and Pompelli, 1987, p. 455) also stress the importance of social variables in understanding alcohol abuse. As Heien and Pompelli (1987, p. 455) found, their results "highlight the importance of sociological factors and downplay the distribution of control variables."

Colón (1979, pp. 93-94) also found that consumption did not predict alcoholism rates. This suggests the significance of diet, body weight, genetics, drinking patterns, cultural expectations and other factors in alcoholism and other drinking problems. It destroys a basic assumption central and essential to the control of consumption model: that drinking problems are closely and directly related to per capita consumption of alcohol.

SOCIO-CULTURAL MODEL IS SUPERIOR

Given the problematic nature of control-of-consumption strategies, their often counter-productive consequences and the moral and ethical difficulties raised by their imposition on non-abusers, it is essential that alternative strategies be sought. The socio-cultural approach, based on the analysis of drinking practices around the world, provides such strategies. It would reinforce those drinking practices that promote responsible moderate drinking and discourage those that discourage such drinking. This approach "may be achieved without impinging upon the freedom of either individual drinkers or abstainers. A policy of both encouraging and discouraging certain types of drinking would leave ample room for individual choice" (Plaut, 1967, p. 125).

Parents who wish their children to drink as adults should both serve as good role models and teach their children gradually how to drink responsibly. If parents wish their children to abstain as adults, they also need to serve as appropriate role models and they need to help their children to develop the attitudes and skills needed to live successfully in a predominately drinking society.

RECOMMENDATIONS

From socio-cultural analyses and scientific evidence flow specific policy recommendations:

I.   The first recommendation is that the current control-of-consumption attack upon alcohol should be terminated.   There exists much evidence that this negative approach to alcohol problems is based on questionable assumptions (e.g., Lauderdale, 1977, pp. 3-5; Colón, 1979, pp. 11-12; Pittman, 1980, p. 44; Skog, 1973, p. 10; Duffy and Cohen, 1978; Parker and Harman, 1978; Duffy, 1978; Alanko, 1992, pp. 3-5), that its policies fail to achieve their objectives (e.g., Graves, 1992, pp. 14-15; Rabow and Watts, 1982; Harford et al., 1979; Ogborne and Smart, 1980, p. 295; Moskowitz, 1989, p. 60; Atkin, 1987, p. 273; Smart, 1982, p. 235; Colón, 1979, pp. 101-102), and that its policies may be counterproductive (e.g., Parker and Harman, 1979, p. 78; Dull and Giacopassi, 1986, pp. 518-519; Popham et al., 1976; Colón, 1982-1983; Linsky et al., 1986; Engs and Hanson, 1989).

II.   The second recommendation is that all attempts to stigmatize beverage alcohol as a "dirty drug," as a poison, as inherently harmful or as a substance to be abhorred and shunned should be terminated.   Alcohol is neither a poison nor a magic elixir capable of solving life's problems.

The place of alcohol in American society has long been ambivalent (Pittman, 1991, p. 776; Mecca, 1980, pp. 4-6; Christie, 1974, p. 9). "Drinking has been blessed and cursed, has been held the cause of economic catastrophe and the hope for prosperity, the major cause of crime, disease and military defeat, depravity and a sign of high prestige, mature personality, and a refined civilization" (Straus and Bacon, 1953). This ambivalence, which has been described as an extreme love-hate relationship (Milgram, 1990, p. 27), is highly undesirable and has negative consequences: "The emotionalism and special meanings assigned to drinking increase the possibility of feelings of guilt, conflict, and anxiety becoming associated with the use of alcohol. They make drinking a readily available focus for psychological problems. This is less likely to happen when drinking is not so endowed with confused, hostile, and frequently concealed emotions."

Stigmatizing alcohol serves no practical purpose, contributes to cultural emotionalism and ambivalence, and exacerbates the problems it seeks to solve.

In stigmatizing alcohol, control proponents may inadvertently trivialize the use of illegal drugs and thereby encourage their use. Or, especially among younger students, they may create the false impression that parents who use alcohol in moderation are drug abusers whose good example they should reject. Thus, their misguided effort to equate alcohol with illicit drugs is likely to be counterproductive.

III. The third recommendation is "That the President of the United States direct the secretary of Health and Human Services, the director of the Alcohol, Drug Abuse and Mental Health Administration and the director of the National Institute for Alcohol Abuse and Alcoholism to formulate and carry out new policies that incorporate the concept of responsible or moderate drinking along with the choice of abstinence" (Ford, 1988, p. 299).

This directive should also apply to the Secretary of the United States Department of Education.

IV. The fourth recommendation is that systematic efforts be made to "Clarify and emphasize the distinctions between acceptable drinking and unacceptable drinking" (Plaut, 1967, p. 142). We need to develop a greater consensus on what constitutes acceptable and unacceptable drinking. "The careful spelling out of what constitutes socially acceptable drinking will be far more difficult than reaching agreement on what types of drinking are to be avoided. The absurdity of defining only 'bad' drinking is analogous to teaching a youngster how to drive only by pointing out what *not* to do . . ." (Plaut, 1967, pp. 142-143, emphasis in original). Young people clearly desire such guidance (Hance, 1981, pp. 81-84).

V. The fifth recommendation is that unacceptable drinking behaviors should be strongly sanctioned, both legally and socially. Importantly, intoxication must not be accepted as an excuse for otherwise unacceptable behavior.

While the criminal justice system has a significant role to play, the most important role must be played by individual peers--friends, relatives, loved ones, co-workers, and other significant others--who assume personal responsibility. "In the long run, the success of efforts to curb drunkenness and other forms of destructive behavior depends on the willingness of Americans to express their concern and take appropriate action when such drinking occurs" (Plaut, 1967, p. 146).

VI. The sixth recommendation is that parents should be permitted to serve alcohol to their offspring of any age, not only in the home, but in restaurants, parks and other locations under their direct control and supervision (Wilkinson, 1970, p. 105).

If parents wish their children to abstain as adults, they need to serve as appropriate role models and to teach them the attitudes and skills they will need in a predominantly drinking society. However, if they wish their children to drink in moderation as adults then they, too, need to serve as appropriate role models and to teach them the appropriate attitudes and skills to drink in moderation.

Cisin (1978, p. 154) has observed:

In our roles as parents and educators, we have responsibility for the socialization of our children, a responsibility for preparing them for life in the world. Part of our job is teaching children how to handle dangerous activities like driving, swimming, drinking, and sex. We behave toward our children as though there were really two different kinds of dangerous activities. Driving and swimming fall into the first type: we carefully teach our children that these are dangerous activities, and we deliberately set out to be sure that they know there is a right way and a wrong way to participate in these activities.

On the other hand, when we look at the other kind of dangerous activities, exemplified by drinking and sex, we seem to know only one word: 'Don't.' We do not bother to say there is a right way and there is a wrong way; we just say 'Don't!' We do not really want to produce abstainers; we have the illusion that they will follow our advice and be abstainers (in the case of sex, until marriage; and in the case of alcohol, until maturity) until they reach the magic age at which they can handle these activities. But as to the rights and wrongs of handling it when the great day comes, we choose to keep them in the dark. Now this is sheer hypocrisy. We are slowly awakening to the fact that we owe our children sex education in the home and in the school--education not dominated by the antisex league. We should be brave enough to tell them the truth; that drinking is normal behavior in the society, that moderate drinking need not lead to abuse; that drinking can be done in an appropriate civilized way without shame and guilt. Perhaps greater socialization in the direction of moderate drinking is part of the program we need for prevention of alcohol problems in the future.

VII. The seventh recommendation is that educational efforts should encourage moderate use of alcohol among those who choose to drink. Such efforts should present moderation in drinking rather than drinking per se as a sign of maturity (Wilkinson, 1970, p. 105).

Alcohol can confer neither adulthood nor masculinity. Unfortunately, a common " . . . cause of trouble is the belief that an ability to 'hold one's liquor' is a sign of manliness; in many circles heavy drinking is equated with masculinity. This belief encourages the drinking of large amounts of alcohol and promotes drunkenness. Because of this linkage of drinking with masculinity, some adolescents and young men (and perhaps older men as well) choose this readily available and generally approved way of demonstrating to themselves and others that they 'really are men'" (Plaut, 1967, p. 130).

It is important that educational efforts present moderate drinking and abstinence as equally acceptable or appropriate choices. And just as those who choose to drink should not force alcohol upon abstainers, "those who choose not to drink alcohol should not attempt to impose that decision or the values surrounding the decision on others" (Education Commission of the States, n.d., p. 4).

CONTROL-OF-CONSUMPTION APPROACH SHOULD BE REJECTED

It has been stressed (Room, 1984, p. 312) that "[c]ontrols that do not have genuine popular consent are likely to be at least partly subverted . . . [and can even have] strongly contrary effects." Peele (1989, p.67) has also quoted Room's (1984, p. 312) observation that "[c]olonial restrictions on alcohol for native populations have left an aftermath of symbolic identification of drinking with personal emancipation . . . [while] rationing schemes in Sweden and Greenland seem to have ended with a kind of national binge."

Similarly, Australian laws closing bars at six o'clock got the working men out of the establishments and possibly home to their families in time for dinner. However, they also produced the undesirable custom known as the six o'clock swill, which involves consuming as much beer as possible between the end of work and the six o'clock closing time (Room, 1976). Sterne and her colleagues (1967) concluded that minimum age laws not only fail in their intent but also produce very questionable consequences.

As indicated in the Introduction, it has been said that if there is one universal characteristic that pervades humanity, it may be the urge to manipulate and control the behavior of others (Cisin, 1978) and "Regardless of how often is fails or leads us in destructive directions, the search for simple solutions to complex problems seems endlessly appealing" (Lazar and Ford, 1977, p. 29). Nowhere is this more apparent than in the control-of-consumption program of questionable legislation to restrict the consumption of alcohol. Like the prohibitionists earlier in the century, whom they so closely resemble, the neo-drys of today are convinced that they have found the solution to reducing alcohol problems. Unfortunately, what we need are not more control-of-consumption laws but the wisdom and courage to move beyond such simplistic answers to a complex social problem.

REFERENCES

Alanko, Timo. Per Capita Consumption and rate of Heavy Use of Alcohol: On Evidence and Inference in the Single Distribution Debate. Paper presented at the Annual Alcohol Epidemiology Symposium of the Kettil Bruuh Society for Social and Epidemiological Research on Alcohol. Toronto, Ontario, May 30 - June 5, 1992.

Asbury, Herbert. *The Great Illusion: An Informal History of Prohibition.* New York: Doubleday & Co., 1950.

Atkin, Charles K. Alcoholic-Beverage Advertising: Its Content and Impact. In: Holder, Harold D. and Mello, Nancy K. (eds.) *Control Issues in Alcohol Abuse Prevention: Strategies for States and Communities.* Greenwich, CT: JAI Press, 1987. pp. 267-

303.

Bacon, Margaret, and Jones, Mary B. *Teen-Age Drinking*. New York: Thomas Y. Crowell, 1968.

Bruun, Kettil. *Drinking Behavior in Small Groups: An Experimental Study*. Helsinki, Finland: Finnish Foundation for Alcohol Studies, 1959.

Christie, Nils. Goals, Ethics and Politics of Preventing Alcohol Problems. In: Room, Robin and Sheffield, Susan (eds.) *The Prevention of Alcohol Problems: Report of a Conference*. Sacramento, CA: Office of Alcoholism, Health and Welfare, 1974. pp. 2-11.

Cisin, Ira H. Formal and Informal Social Control over Drinking. In: Ewing, John A. and Rouse, Beatrice A. (eds.) *Drinking: Alcohol in American Society - Issues and Current Research*. Chicago, IL: Nelson-Hall, 1978. pp. 145-158.

Colón, Israel. Alcohol Control Policies and their Relation to Alcohol Consumption and Alcoholism. Unpublished Ph.D. dissertation, Brandeis University, 1979.

Colón, Israel. The influence of state monopoly of alcohol distribution and the frequency of package stores on single motor vehicle fatalities. *American Journal of Drug and Alcohol Abuse*, 1982-1983, *9*, 315-331.

de Lint, Jan. Recent trends in Dutch drinking. A problem case for availability explanations. *Contemporary Drug Problems*, 1981, *10*, 179-192.

Duffy, John C. Comment on "The single distribution theory of alcohol consumption" *Journal of Studies on Alcohol*, 1978, *39*, 1648-1650.

Duffy, John C., and Cohen, G. R. Total alcohol consumption and excessive drinking. *British Journal of Addiction*, 1978, *73*, 259-264.

Dull, R. Thomas and Giacopassi, David J. An assessment of the effects of alcohol ordinances on selected behaviors and conditions. *The Journal of Drug Issues*, 1986, *16*, 511-521.

Education Commission of the States. Task Force on Responsible Decision about Alcohol. *Final Report*. Denver, CO: Education Commission of the States. Task Force on Responsible Decisions about Alcohol, Booklet Number 2, n.d.

Engelmann, Larry. *Intemperance: The Lost War Against Liquor*. New York: Free Press, 1979.

Engs, Ruth C., and Hanson, David J. Reactance theory: A test with collegiate drinking. *Psychological Reports*, 1989, *64*, 1083-1086.

Engs, Ruth C., and Hanson, David J. Boozing and brawling on campus: A national study of violent problems associated with drinking over the past decade. *Journal of Criminal Justice*, 1994, *22*, 171-180.

Everest, Allan S. *Rum Across the Border: The Prohibition Era in Northern New York*. Syracuse, NY: Syracuse University Press, 1978.

Ewing, John A., and Rouse, Beatrice A. Drinks, drinkers, and drinking. In: Ewing, John A., and Rouse, Beatrice A. (eds.) *Drinking: Alcohol in American Society - Issues and Current Research*. Chicago, IL: Nelson-Hall, 1976. pp. 5-30.

Fallding, Harold. *Drinking, Community and Civilization*. New Brunswick, NJ: Rutgers Center of Alcohol Studies, 1974.

Ford, Gene. *The Benefits of Moderate Drinking: Alcohol, Health and Society*. San Francisco, CA: Wine Appreciation Guild, 1988.

Goldberg, Steven. Putting Science in the Constitution: The Prohibition Experience. In: Kyvig, David E. (ed.) *Law, Alcohol, and Order: Perspectives on National Prohibition*. Westport, CT: Greenwood Press, 1985. pp. 21-34.

Grant, Marcus and Ritson, Bruce. *Alcohol: The Prevention Debate.* New York: St. Martin's Press, 1983.

Graves, Karen L. Do Warning Labels on Alcoholic Beverages Make a Difference? A Comparison of the United States and Ontario, Canada between 1990 and 1991. Paper presented at the Annual Alcohol Epidemiology Symposium of the Kettil Bruun Society for Social and Epidemiological Research on Alcohol. Toronto, Ontario, May 30 - June 5, 1992.

Gross, Leonard. *How Much is too Much?: The Effects of Social Drinking.* New York: Random House, 1983.

Hance, Emilie S. Teenage Drinking in San Francisco. Unpublished M.A. thesis, San Francisco State University, 1981.

Harford, Thomas C., Parker, Douglas A., Paulter, Charles, and Wolz, Michael. Relationship between the number of on-premise outlets and alcoholism. *Journal of Studies on Alcohol,* 1979, *40,* 1053-1057.

Heath, Dwight B. A decade of development in the anthropological study of alcohol use: 1970-1980. In: Douglas, Mary (ed.) *Constructive Drinking: Perspectives on Drink from Anthropology.* Cambridge University Press, 1987. pp. 16-69.

Heien, Dale and Pompelli, Greg. Stress, ethnic and distribution factors in a dichotomous response model of alcohol abuse. *Journal of Studies on Alcohol,* 1987, *48,* 450-455.

Hilton, Michael E. and Clark, Walter B. Changes in American drinking patterns and problems, 1967-1984. *Journal of Studies on Alcohol,* 1987, *48,* 515-522.

Kobler, John. *Ardent Spirits: The Rise and Fall of Prohibition.* New York: G. P. Putnam's Sons, 1973.

Lauderdale, Michael L. *An Analysis of the Control Theory of Alcoholism.* Denver, CO: Education Commission of the States, 1977.

Lazar, Irving and Ford, John. Untitled reaction of review panel. In: Lauderdale, Michael L. *An Analysis of the Control Theory of Alcoholism.* Denver, CO: Education Commission of the States, 1977. pp. 29-34.

Levine, Harry G. Temperance and Women in 19th-Century United States. In: Kalant, Oriana J. (ed.) *Alcohol and Drug Problems in Women: Research Advances in Alcohol and Drug Problems.* Vol. 5. New York: Plenum, 1980. pp. 25-67.

Linsky, Arnold S., Colby, Jr., John P., and Straus, Murray A. Drinking norms and alcohol-related problems in the United States. *Journal of Studies on Alcohol,* 1986, *47,* 384-393.

MacAndrew, Craig, and Edgerton, Robert. *Drunken Comportment: A Social Explanation.* Chicago, IL: Aldine, 1969.

Maine State Department of Education. Leadership in Maine. Augusta, ME: Maine State Department of Education n.d. (Poster)

Mäkelä, Klaus. Level of Consumption and Social Consequences of Drinking. In: Israel, Yedy, Glaser, Frederick B., Kalant, Harold, Popham, Robert E., Schmidt, Wolfgang, Smart, Reginald G. (eds.) *Research Advances in Alcohol and Drug Problems,* Volume 4. New York, Plenum Press, 1978. pp. 303-348.

Mandelbaum, David G. Alcohol and Culture. In: Marshall, Mac (ed.) *Beliefs, Behaviors, & Alcoholic Beverages: A Cross-Cultural Survey.* Ann Arbor, MI: University of Michigan Press, 1979, pp. 14-30. Reprinted from *Current Anthropology,* 1965, *6,* No. 3, 281-293.

Marlatt, G. Alan and Rohsenow, Damaris J. The think-drink effect. *Psychology Today,* 1981, *15,* 60-69, 93.

Marshall, Mac. Conclusions. In: Marshall, Mac (ed.) *Beliefs, Behaviors, & Alcoholic Beverages: A Cross-Cultural Survey.* Ann Arbor, MI: University of Michigan Press, 1979. pp. 451-458.

Mecca, Andrew M. *Alcoholism in America: A Modern Perspective.* Belvedere, CA: California Health Research Foundation, 1980.

Milgram, Gail G. *The Facts about Drinking.* Mount Vernon, NY: Consumers Union, 1990.

Moskowitz, Joel M. The primary prevention of alcohol problems: A critical review of the research literature. *Journal of Studies on Alcohol,* 1989, *50,* 54-88.

Ogborne, Alan C., and Smart, Reginald G. Will restrictions on alcohol advertising reduce alcohol consumption? *British Journal of Addiction,* 1980, *75,* 293-296.

Parker, Douglas A. and Harman, Marsha S. A Critique of the Distribution of Consumption Model of Prevention. In: Harford, Thomas C. and Parker, Douglas A. (eds.) *Normative Approaches to the Prevention of Alcohol Abuse and Alcoholism.* Rockville, MD: National Institute on Alcohol Abuse and Alcoholism, 1979. pp. 67-88.

Peele, Stanton. *Diseasing of America: Addiction Treatment out of Control.* Lexington, MA: Lexington Books, 1989.

Pittman, David J. *Primary Prevention of Alcohol Abuse and Alcoholism: An Evaluation of the Control of Consumption Policy.* St. Louis, MO: Washington University, Social Science Institute, 1980.

Pittman, David J. The New Temperance Movement. In: Pittman, David J. and White, Helene R. (ed.) *Society, Culture, and Drinking Patterns Reexamined.* New Brunswick, NJ: Rutgers Center of Alcohol Studies, 1991. pp. 775-790.

Plaut, Thomas F. A. *Alcohol Problems: A Report to the Nation by the Cooperative Commission on the Study of Alcoholism.* New York: Oxford University Press, 1967.

Popham, Robert E. The Social History of the Tavern. In: Israel, Yedy, Glaser, Frederick B., Kalant, Harold, Popham, Robert E., Schmidt, Wolfgang, and Smart, Reginald G. (eds.) *Research Advances in Alcohol and Drug Problems.* Vol. 4. New York: Plenum, 1978. pp. 225-302.

Popham, Robert, Schmidt, Wolgang, and de Lint, Jan. The Effect of Legal Restraint on Drinking. In: Kissin, Benjamin, and Begleiter, Henri (eds.) *Social Aspects of Alcoholism.* New York: Plenum Press, Vol. 4, 1976. pp. 579-625.

Rabow, Jerome, and Watts, Ronald K. Alcohol availability, alcoholic beverage sales and alcohol-related problems. *Journal of Studies on Alcohol,* 1982, *43,* 767-801.

Room, Robin. Alcohol control and public health. *Annual Review of Public Health,* 1984, *5,* 293-317.

Room, Robin. Evaluating the Effect of Drinking Laws on Drinking. In: Ewing, John A. and Rouse, Beatrice A. (eds.) *Drinking: Alcohol in American Society - Issues and Current Research.* Chicago, IL: Nelson-Hall, 1976. pp. 267-289.

Rorabaugh, William. *The Alcoholic Republic.* New York: Oxford University Press, 1979.

Sinclair, Andrew. *Prohibition: The Era of Excess.* Boston: Little, Brown and Co., 1962.

Skog, Ole-Jørgen. Less alcohol--fewer alcoholics? *The Drinking and Drug Practices Surveyor,* 1973, No. 7, 7-13.

Smart, Reginald G. The Impact of Prevention Measures: An Examination of Research Findings. In: Institute of Medicine. *Legislative Approaches to Prevention of Alcohol-*

Related Problems: An Inter-American Workshop-Proceedings. Washington, DC: National Academy Press, 1982. pp. 224-246.

Smith, C. J. The wrath of grapes: The health-related implications of changing American drinking practices. *Area*, 1985, 97-108.

Sterne, M. W., Pittman, D. J. and Coe, T. Teenagers, Drinking and the Law: Study of Arrest Trends for Alcohol-Related Offenses. In: Pittman, David J. (ed.) *Alcoholism.* New York: Harper and Row, 1967. pp. 55-56.

Straus, Robert and Bacon, Selden D. *Drinking in College.* New Haven, CT: Yale University Press, 1953.

Strayton, W. H. Our experiment in national Prohibition. What progress has it made? *Annals of the American Academy of Political and Social Science*, 1923, *109*, 26-38.

Sulkunen, P. Drinking Patterns and the Level of Alcohol Consumption: An International Overview. In: Gibbins, R. J., Israel, Yedy, Kalant, Harold, Popham, Robert E., Schmidt, Wolfgang, and Smart, Reginald G. (eds.) *Research Advances in Alcohol and Drug Problems*, Volume 3. New York: John Wiley & Sons, 1976. pp. 223-281.

Wilkinson, Rupert. *The Prevention of Drinking Problems: Alcohol Control and Cultural Influences.* New York: Oxford University Press, 1970.

Zinberg, Norman E., and Fraser, Kathleen M. The role of the social setting in the prevention and treatment of alcoholism. In: Mendelson, Jack H. and Mello, Nancy K. (eds.) *The Diagnosis and Treatment of Alcoholism.* New York: McGraw-Hill, second edition, 1985. pp. 457-483.

Author Index

Subject Index

About the Author

DAVID J. HANSON is Professor of Sociology and Director of Assessment at the State University of New York at Potsdam. He has written over 270 works—journal articles and books on this or related topics.

ISBN 0-275-94926-5

EAN

HARDCOVER BAR CODE